What others are saying –

Arif Ahmad's *A Piece of Me* is an original and provocative mixed genre work that blends poetry with prose, memoirs and political op-eds. Ahmad's writing reflects his myriad experiences as a physician committed to the hard task of saving lives. Juxtaposed against Ahmad's vocation of interventional cardiology is the random violence of the world, acts of mass shooting in the U.S. and religious extremism elsewhere. The book is a negotiation of Ahmad's identity as a Muslim immigrant physician in a post 9/11 America grappling with extremes of political polarization. Ahmad displays remarkable openness and compassion in trying to make sense of rising intolerance. The most moving parts of the book remain those rare insights into his personal struggles, the illness and care of his father, the memory of the tragic loss of his brother, his personal pilgrimage to Mecca, and his commitment above all to peaceful co-existence in the U.S. and the world. This is an important work voicing the complex experiences of an often silenced and misunderstood minority.

Lopamudra Basu, Ph.D.
Professor of English
University of Wisconsin-Stout.

....

There is a time travel of sensitive, apt and preemptive validation of reality through these writings, *A Piece of Me*.

Most impressive is the way you have expressed the emotion of patriotic values such as equality, women empowerment, rejecting discrimination, hope, and peace while creating American identity from the perspective of our diaspora.

The writing is eloquent, creative and is an active voice that draws us into an emotion of collective expression. The two pearls in the string of beautiful pearls that stand out are the ones that you dedicated to your parents and your daughter. No wonder resilience and optimism depicts in every step of your journey.

Dr. Lubna Naeem,
San Antonio, TX

....

Being a good observer and listener make Arif an excellent writer. His work across multiple disciplines broadly addresses the narrative of human experience.

By artfully putting complex thoughts and ideas into simple and clear language using a robust vocabulary, Arif powerfully addresses human conflicts both without and within. He describes the human condition based on inequality of gender, race, and religion and his writings always leave a strong impression.

Dr. Shakaib Razzaq,
Milwaukee, WI

....

A PIECE OF ME by Arif Ahmad is a must-read for anyone who is a protagonist of treating people with kindness regardless of race, gender, and religion.

The book is an album of poetic well-versed essays of commentary, perspective, and opinions of Ahmad on diverse challenges facing our humanity. At first glance, the essays seem embedded unceremoniously, but they slowly but surely engage the reader and steadily tend to hold one's interest.

It's a mantra of affirmations that time will tell are symbolic or have any practical effect. Personally, I loved reading this book.

Dr. Ayub Khawaja,
Lahore, Pakistan

....

I felt I was exploring through the eyes and heart of another. What a joy it has been to read this collection, some poetry – some prose and to feel such heartfelt emotions. While not shying away from some of America's most contentious challenges, Dr. Arif Ahmad, a Pakistani American cardiologist, has a way of bringing things to life, not condemning us but just questioning how things are, or how we all hope someday they will be.

By openly exploring our 'separateness' of color and religion, he has transcended that same separateness by 'lighting the path of oneness' in our glorious pursuit of peace.

C. Susan Nunn
Author, Editor and Writing Coach

A PIECE OF ME

*an arrangement of words to
inspire reflection*

Arif Ahmad

July 2021, *A Piece of Me*

All rights reserved. No part of this publication may be reproduced, distributed, or transmitted in any form by any means, including photocopying, recording, or other electronic methods without the prior written permission of the author, except in the case of brief quotations embodied in reviews and certain other noncommercial uses permitted by copyright law. For permission requests, write to the author at the address below.

Arif Ahmad
RF publishing, LLC
rfpublishing1@gmail.com

ISBN:
   978-1-7373929-0-3 Amazon Kindle eBook
   978-1-7373929-1-0 Amazon Paperback

Printed in the United States of America
First Printing, July 2021

Dedication

For my mother, wife, and daughter

FOREWORD

My dad often says, "the enemy of good is better."

He doesn't much believe in micro-analyzing and over-editing himself, mostly because of his surety in being good. In many ways, he is good. But not perfect. And that's okay.

Anytime he would ask me or my brother how something sounded, a certain line or the flow of word choice, he was pretty sure he wasn't going to make any edits regardless of what we said because he knows his writing better than anyone. He knows it rarely ever needs much, if any, work. Much of that has to do with natural talent, but a good part of it comes from him being able to set solid, respectable standards for himself that he consistently meets.

He's incredibly passionate about his writing, and it shows. For someone who most would consider keeps to himself, he's incredibly expressive and loud with his written word.

I like writing too, so much so that I've made it my profession, unlike my dad. He's made writing one of his favorite pastimes. I'm a journalist, though, so the difference also is that I write plainly as a realist while my dad writes as a realist who skews towards optimism.

My dad rarely expresses his stress. He often stays in his own world, in his own head, with a million things swirling around. When something is pressing on his mind enough, he prefers to talk it through. Oftentimes, it's something pressing only to him. But he'll never actually say that something is troubling him.

A Piece of Me

I think this is partly because of his faith in everything working out, that everything will be okay. His optimism and his faith go hand in hand. Because he is a man of faith, he knows however busy he gets, however tense the times get, stress is only temporary and better times are always on the horizon.

Something my dad and I have in common when it comes to our writing is that we aren't limited to one subject or topic area. I'm a general assignment reporter, which means I write about pretty much anything at any time, depending on what's needed and what's happening. I find a lot of joy in doing so because it keeps things interesting, and it keeps me on my toes. My dad also writes about anything and everything. He doesn't limit himself, his ideas, opinions or otherwise.

He shares his thoughts on politics, culture, humanity, life, death and beyond, always with a recurring theme of hopefulness. He shares his perspectives as a Muslim and a Pakistani immigrant in the United States, a physician, and an avid outdoorsman. In this book, he's compiled these pieces of himself and more. And that's what you'll truly get. Pieces of himself, not anyone else or some version of himself. It's not perfect, but it's always good.

Shanzeh Ahmad

INTRODUCTION

What might a Muslim, Pakistani American Physician have to say about the decade that was?

For a private person, *A Piece of Me* feels like baring the most intimate realms of my soul. Some of my writings have followed the ebb of time and are reactionary, while others are time-independent.

I grew up in Lahore, Pakistan. Studying at Sacred Heart and Saint Anthony's gave me a global perspective early on. A Ravian (Government College) and an Iqbalian (Allama Iqbal Medical College) followed. I came to the USA in 1993 to train and practice in Internal Medicine, Cardiology, and Electrophysiology.

American Midwest is home, and the Muslim faith is how I know of reaching for the Divine. To become a better Samaritan is a challenge I keep at.

Because I have worked hard and sacrificed much, I cherish, enjoy, and am rather protective of the strengths that brought me to America. All this and more inspire me to write boldly both in word and thought and often with an optimistic twist and in a form I call my own.

I use the written word to emote, often untamed and exact out of my heart. The rhythm of my words is inspired by the Quran and the writings of Sir Allama Iqbal.

Multiple Board Certified, I am a Fellow of American College of Cardiology and a Fellow of Heart Rhythm Society. My profession, family, friends, and the outdoors are my passion and something I live for.

CONTENTS

Your Average Muslim Joe and Mary 1
What Muslims, Ahmad Who 2
Once There Was this Mr. Man 3
I Keep Trying 4
You Greedy Me 5
See This Happening 6
A People 7
A Place Called "Nowhere" 8
Almost Equal 9
It is Time 10
I Often Wonder 11
American Shame 12
Hope 13
Barack Hussein Obama 15
Death of Decency 16
Who I Really am 17
To Whom It May Concern 18
This I Believe 19
Catch my Plea 20
The Optimist 22
Where are the Mandelas, The Gandhis of this Century? 23

Francis, you Beauty	25
You Go Girl	27
Yara	28
Why	30
Who are you, and What are you Made of?	31
Welcome Home	32
Us Muslims	34
Trump's Red Hot Middle America and Here is Why	35
To Appna	37
Tip of the Iceberg	39
Those Mile-Long Chevrolets	40
Think it Over any Which Way	41
The Workout	42
July 2020	44
The Reset	45
Early in the Pandemic	47
The Girl of My Dreams	48
The American Gun Law Paradox	50
Take a Knee	51
Struggle	53
State of Pakistan	54
Reality Check	55
As an American Muslim	57
President Obama's Reply	59
Prez O	60
Please	61

Pink 64

Paris, January 7th, 2015 65

Pakistan Zindabad (Long Live Pakistan) 66

Pain 69

Optimism on the Ropes 70

One Earth, One Species 71

One and One 72

On our Very Own 73

Of I and Me 75

News 76

No Need for Election Reforms in Appna 77

Nation of Similar Only 78

The Inspiration That is an American President 80

Our Beloved Appna 82

My Jesus Moment 84

My Brother 85

My Apology 87

Music Out of a Physician's Keyboard 89

"Me Too" of a Different Kind 92

Dear God the Grievance and the Response 94

My Dear Creation "The Response" 96

Mandela 98

Making of a False Fact 100

Mainstream American Media 101

The Main Draw in this Cosmos 103

Love this Pain 104

Lota in Chicago	105
Look Pretty Living	107
Land of the Pure	108
Jai	109
Istanbul	111
In our Cities of Today	114
I Love the Fourteenth of August	116
Hello Silver	117
Americans are Pitted Against one Another	118
Hajj, Go for it	119
Golden Embolden	124
Golden age	126
God and Inclusiveness	132
Fundamentally one	134
From Behind the Mask	135
Fresh Tracks	136
For the Sake of Heavens, for Heaven's Sake	137
For all its Criticism	139
Enough	140
Distracted	141
Dear Mr. Donald Trump	143
Children will be Children	145
But Wait A Second	146
Bosa of Hajr-E-Aswad (Kissing of the Black Stone)	147
An Atypical Pitch to Exercise	151
Boo	153

Coming Together is on You, Me, and Everyone 154

Aylan 156

Appna Perfect 157

Appna Elections 2017 159

American Joker. 160

American Afghan War Surge and Pakistan Bashing 161

America's Gun Violence, A Curse, or God's Retribution? 164

America you Beauty 165

America is its People. 167

A Very American Thing 168

A Gift, Early in the Pandemic 169

38-Year-Old Jacinda Ardern, A Messiah and A Woman 170

32 Expatriates, Pakistanis, and Indians Against a Nuclear Standoff . . . 171

1.8 Billion Villains 172

YOUR AVERAGE MUSLIM JOE AND MARY

(April 2015, at a time when the majority of Muslims were caught in the crossfire)

Eradicated en masse by the Muslim fundamentalists for not being Muslim enough and siding with the West.

Tried unilaterally in the media, embarrassed, condemned, regarded with suspicion, frisked at the airports, many having lost their lives and checked off as collateral damage by the warring West.

Often misunderstood and taken out of context.

Never for a conflict, we like it quiet and out of the limelight.

Not expecting anyone to bail us out or elevate our status.

Some fault for all this surely lies with us.

We are your average Muslim Joe and Mary, the single largest casualty, the silent tragedy of this war on terror.

And it is for us to find a way out of this rut.

To become a world-class scientist, a politician, an artist, an entrepreneur, a philosopher.

Excel at living and never say never.

WHAT MUSLIMS, AHMAD WHO

(September 2017,
better thyself and better this World)

Positive achievements by a large group of people in a broad sense, yes.

Christians can take credit for the Modern World, the West.

Hindus have a rising India to boast of.

Jews, fewer in numbers, hold sway over finance and media.

Atheists govern the powerhouse that is China.

Now show me some positives, a positive, we Muslims have on display.

1.7 billion is only a number.

Some oil-rich Gulf States, as if having oil is a measure of performance.

What else, still thinking, am I missing anything?

Bits and pieces people, what is our mutual claim to fame?

Soul searching or shifting the blame?

What is our best foot forward?

Not self-combustion, backstabbing, and terrorism.

We total less than the sum of our parts.

Thus, I'm not getting used to being called out and kicked around.

When one more time, we can turn out excited, brilliant, and proud.

Only how?

ONCE THERE WAS THIS MR. MAN

(March 2020, early in the Pandemic)

once there was this Mr. Man
yes, you are, and I am
demigods losing the plot
chuckle before you read this
done in by a tiny covid

19
who let you in
besides oceans and walls
alien pathogen
this country is for our citizens
you just ain't welcome

Mr. Man says the virus
you're your worst nemesis
for a small me
do you even see
the tall lessons

top economies now on their knees
if panic and fear were solutions
this by now would be behind us
the unusual times urge our kind
pull together, think others
revise our priorities and relevance

Yours sincerely,
from the frontlines

I KEEP TRYING

(December 2019)

I keep trying harder and harder
adding one wrong to another
piling mine over theirs
hoping that
come a day they might
add up to become a right

YOU GREEDY ME

(January 2017, as a cry to Mr. Schindler,
this time to save a Muslim soul from persecution)

Take me on your list
1200 plus 1 or the one
This never warring child of Abraham
This ahmad, arif, remember
As you grow more relevant
One more time
Dear Mr. Schindler

SEE THIS HAPPENING

(September 2017)

Come with me on a mental exercise.
Give me the best way of bringing down a nation?
Take America, for example.
How can America be defeated?
Not by force against the World's best military.
Not monetarily upon the World's largest economy.
No, it cannot be politically isolated.
Still, there is a way, a very smart one at that.
Polarize and divide them Americans.
Have them hate each other, choke them, create doubt.
Pitch people against people, let America defeat itself.
Do from within, which cannot be done from without.

A PEOPLE

(October 2018)

In celebration of our differences
Craving for more respect, more relevance
All before self
Deep-rooted yet visible
In him, her and all
Knocking, piercing, screaming
This urge, the roar, the calling
A conviction to carve a Nation
Our will is to become a People

A PLACE CALLED "NOWHERE"

(May 2014)

Our minds clueless and hearts of stone
With eyes wide shut
We aim at each other in the dark
Hoping to come close and bridge the gap
For every two steps forward
We take three back
Stuck in this fool's paradise
and hoping to arrive
At the lofty peaks of love
Which cannot sustain life
Where there is no air
It is right there
Here
This City of Peace
A place called "Nowhere"

ALMOST EQUAL

(August 2017, praying for equality)

This game, we were playing making faces at each other
Except I was the one to end up on the altar
Turns out that with my name,
I should not have been playing this game
And also, that I was a shade too dark
I tug on my freedoms before I write
Please God, please
In another life, let me be blond, blue-eyed, and white

IT IS TIME

(August 2016, US elections, a woman in the lead,
I wrote this for my daughter on her birthday)

Discrimination is alive and well.

Against minorities, on religious, racial, and social lines, sexual preferences, and gender orientation.

This one, however, remains astonishing for its persistence and the sheer numbers.

Prejudice against half of this world's population.

That against Women.

Subtle or obvious, it remains unrelenting, and in some way, form or shape is always there.

And yes, it is still present in the most sophisticated of the societies.

Be it unequal remuneration or receiving less aggressive medical care.

Or as in still waiting for the first Woman President to lead this planet's most advanced nation.

A wait now for well over two centuries.

Please try and explain this.

As I hope that an American Woman President, the leader of the free world, shall inspire Women everywhere and cut into this bias.

It is time.

I OFTEN WONDER

(February 2017)

As a physician cardiologist, I witness and participate in the drama of life and death every single day, and on my way back from work, I often wonder.

I wonder about the disparity of effort between the acts of saving life and taking life. One is so hard, difficult, and temporary. The other seems so easy, effortless, and permanent.

I wonder about the long, tough hours spent in trying to save a life, to help sustain and better a life, to preserve and heal a life.

I contrast this to life wasted, cut short, and taken away in conflicts and wars, crime, combat, hostilities and aggression, terror, and counter-terror.

Life ended purposefully and without purpose, with vengeance and malice and in the blink of an eye.

Living one moment and dead the next.

The sudden cessation of a beating heart, the gleam in the eyes changing to dull, irreversible, and forever.

I wonder why saving life is so arduous and taking it not so.

And so I stay wondering, I stay working, I keep hoping, and I keep dreaming.

And to those who take life, I say, "For once, try saving one."

AMERICAN SHAME

(Dec 2016, a Muslim Registry
in America is being talked about)

Any more than there already is. I refuse to register. Please don't go there. Incarcerate me instead.

I refuse to discriminate or be discriminated against. I refuse to hate.

I refuse to be a second-rate citizen. Not here, not in this Nation.

I am a Muslim and a person. I refuse to become an American disgrace.

Stir not what cannot be unstirred. Let the psyche stay pure and unperturbed.

Colored yes, tainted yes, unequal yes, I am not a terrorist.

Period.

Condemn an entire people for the actions of a few?

Where in history and the present shall we start and end?

With this, I rest my argument.

HOPE

(April 2016)

Dear Muslim Jihadist,

It feels like yesterday when you accounted for all of them lives, and with your own included.

And I am not here to demonize, patronize or judge you on your motive.

I concede that you may have faced your own provocation and injustice.

But besides your reasons, this is to update you on the state of affairs since.

The religion, yours, mine, ours is in turmoil as we are fighting with and killing most of, and then some more Muslims.

Divided into Shia and Sunni, confused, tentative, defensive are some of the states we are in.

The children of Noah, of Abraham, people of One God, fighting, shedding blood is how the big picture reads.

In some ways, we may have lost the forest for the trees.

So make a wild guess as to what is on the rise.

The non-believers, the agnostics, the atheists,

and I am not sure how thrilled God is with all this.

A Piece of Me

A very rudimentary question in my mind goes as such.

If your loved ones were hurt for no fault of theirs, is harming the no-fault loved ones of others the correct response?

For how is God going to settle between you and your victims?

Many of them were aiming for the very same Heavens.

Still, there is hope as I think of the life of Jesus, or Joseph treating his brothers or Muhammad the Meccans.

And I wonder about your true potential, the could have been.

You were willing to lay your life for a cause.

Only if you could make your point by harnessing those energies for all our well-being.

The rage of hate, revenge, and regress turned into the passion for loving, embrace, and progress.

The kind of stuff legends are made of, yes.

BARACK HUSSEIN OBAMA

(February 2015,
a study of race in America)

A person of color, and you find the going a little rough.

Feel a lot coming at you, some say tough luck.

Now imagine you hold the top office in the world and that you are black.

Welcome to the world of a man they call Barack.

I cannot find a better example of the state of race in 2015 America than this one person.

A man of color called unpatriotic, communist, liar, shown a finger in his face, that he was never a born American.

Not to mention the new curse word, Muslim.

If on the receiving end of all this is the President of the United States, what are the odds stacked against a child of color standing at a street corner?

Yes, when it comes to race in America, we have come a long way and yet have some distance left to cover.

Still, the story here is not what has been hurled at him for the color of his skin.

The story is his response or lack of to all this.

The real story is of inspiration in the mold of Ali, King, and Mandela.

That history would add another name to this distinguished list.

That of Barack Hussein Obama.

For carrying his color and poise the way he did.

DEATH OF DECENCY

(May 2018,
as the rhetoric keeps getting ugly)

I had no idea, the last time I saw her, and she was doing so well. With a capital D swell to the right, followed by an elegant e and a cute little c and then another e, she looked very happy. Little did I know that she was struggling, struggling to be.

Life was so much better with you around, my dear Decency.

WHO I REALLY AM

(September 2016)

From Lahore, Pakistan, which I am.
A Physician, a Muslim, an American.
Only this is a beginning, for I am more.
A piece of you, a part of all denominations.
Our place, its relevance, this canvas.
My reasoning is Earthian. In my mind, the Universe.
We are the World in this as one.
The World is who I really am.

TO WHOM IT MAY CONCERN

(November 2018)

I, me, my, mine
is my predicament
honest, stripped
this is who I am
I can't help it
I am such programmed
thus
disrespected, discounted
bounced around
used for granted
I refuse to realize
the advantage of many
over a few
ever a person
never a nation
then I complain

THIS I BELIEVE

(September 2018)

Such is the nature of this beast that I believe not one conflict of any nature or scale is an unequivocal complete fault of only one side

Not one

And if this premise can be agreed upon

Then therein lies the solution

CATCH MY PLEA

(October 2014)

What is with all "that light"
For just another ordinary day
How in the world can it end this way?
No warning, no nothing
And there I lay
Not breathing
Motionless
A heart gone silent
And "that light"
Oops
Wait
It cannot be
I am not ready
This has to be a mistake
I thought I had time yet
To clean up my act
To wipe off my slate
I've repeatedly wronged myself
A horror show of transgressions,
and a closet load of skeletons,
have been plenty cruel to me
Please
Someone, anyone
Catch my plea
Can I live it over
Do it right, do it better

Arif Ahmad

Try and make amends
Get another chance
Go back once

THE OPTIMIST

(June 2013, dedicated to my mother, Ismat Bano, and
father, Abdul Majeed for teaching me optimism.)

Tough economic times, wars, famine, tsunamis, global meltdown, moral and ethical dehiscence.

So is the glass half-full or half-empty?

Enough going on to sap the energies, to drain the enthusiasm. Enough going on to cloud common sense.

But wait.

It refuses to be a pessimist. It believes in the human will, the human resilience, the human rebound.

It believes in the human race to stand up and deliver.

Every human being to be counted and ask, how can it better another life, how can it make proud mother earth, how can it first do no harm?

It is the good Samaritan, it is the human spirit, it is a dreaming child.

The question is, can it become I, we, us, yet again.

WHERE ARE THE MANDELAS, THE GANDHIS OF THIS CENTURY?

(February 2014, too much killing
for one reason or another)

The pandora box of terrorism and a world spinning on its head
For our choice of dying, which is a better death
From terrorism or as collateral damage
Either way, if you notice
The dead invariably stay dead

Watching, waiting Gods, please look away
Show some patience, hold Your say
Wait till Your judgment day
Unless
We, the chosen ones
You are confusing with angels
Lest You forget
We are not done killing our own
Not just yet

Whatever happened to kindness
The good old goodness
Thoughtfulness
Why is bitter the new norm
Where are the Mandelas, the Gandhis of this century
Fourteen years in, we are waiting, and so is history
Can you step forward and make yourself known
Before we ruin it all, before it's all gone

A Piece of Me

These crazy proxy modern wars
With people dying on all sides
Some not knowing why or for what cause
If killing would make the world safer somehow
Wouldn't this be a very safe planet by now?
If wars were the solution
Where is the "lived happily ever after" conclusion

FRANCIS, YOU BEAUTY

(September 2015)

Just as I had promised myself a break from writing, he shows up
Such inspiration, Oh my God
Is this Pope impressive or what
A Fiat 500 in DC
Washing, kissing feet of people condemned by our society
Women, Children, Muslims included
Seriously
His shoes ordinary black and not the crafted red
His car not a Mercedes but with 190K on it, a 1984 Renault
His living in modest guest house apartments and not the palatial suites
And his love of spending time with the downtrodden at every opportunity
With eyes closed and in my mind only, I imagined, tried, and failed in even imitating such humility
On the side of tears and smiles, this one Pontiff is for the ages
Tolerant and all-inclusive, he talks our language, that of the masses
Mixed in with a lot of common sense
And believes in a singular, common Divine
And asks us to be kind
To each other and to this world
And to them less privileged
He totally totally gets it
That our bigger enemy often is not without but within
That war is the supreme villain
That we partner in this planet's blessings and its sufferings
That when people fight and divide, God often ends up on the losing side
That a nuclear truce is an unclear truce

A Piece of Me

Recommending a "Culture of Care," he is clearly brokering Worldly Peace
Please pretty please
Can we all unite behind him for some days?
For our very sake
Pape
You can be my Pied Piper any day of the week
And so what if I am a Muslim, a Hindu, an Atheist
It is obvious that so many have your ear
Dear Catholics, shall we share him with you for I know it won't bother him a bit

YOU GO GIRL

(December 2016, Malala Yousafzai,
a Pakistani activist for female education
and the youngest Nobel Prize laureate)

Look around hard wherever you are
Do you see the circus of the men, by the men, for the men
In all shades of gray
Egocentric, narcissistic men
Where class act is a handful
And the rest of us just pretend

Dispensable, lesser beings, always second, the inferior sex
Here women are held primarily in a support act
For as and when needed
Though first up in taking our yelling, beating, abuse
Women's lib sounds so romanticizing, so glorifying, so neat
Often, it fails to realize, it struggles to exist

Whichever way you slice it
The pale blue dot remains testosterone-laden
Male-dominated, male-driven
Except
This one girl who may chance to challenge some of this and change some of that
The girl with a facial droop and a reconstructed skull from a bullet that traveled her head
This girl may save us men from us
God willing, Inshallah
You go girl, Malala

YARA

(June 2017)

Out in the wilderness, and this feeling
The rhythm, and this something
All around in them all being
With no beginning,
or end
My own though inevitable, impending

Miracles large and small
Here nothing on show is in my control
So much life so full of life
Silver exuding moon, sun pouring gold
The umpteen shades of green
Smiling for no reason, crazy I ain't

Still that presence
One calming influence
Feel it at times
Besides my weight in sins
Yes
Yara
Bandeya
Bulleya
What is Taqwa?
Is this Khuda?

Footnote:
Khuda is God.
Taqwa is God-consciousness.
Bulleya is Bulleh Shah, a Sufi poet, philosopher of the yesteryears.
Bandeya a person, a creation of the Divine.
Yara is an informal close friend.

WHY

(February 2019)

I don't get it
why we ever remain
only a few
irrelevant
bottom feeders
underachievers
legends of our mind
And we used to enter into vain discourse with those who entered into vain discourses
(Al-Muddathir 45)
in love with I
together
a different story
together
a failure
why?

WHO ARE YOU, AND WHAT ARE YOU MADE OF?

(February 2015)

Yes, you have been wronged
For one reason or the other
Over and over

A brave few took it on, spoke about it
The rest of us, the politically correct, kept our quiet
And that is all right
For therein lies your chance
To rise above the hate, the indifference

Who are you, and what are you made of?

What else are you going to do about it
Stay sorry for yourself, blame everyone under the sun, and buy into the conspiracy theory
Or
Wear your best attitude, bring your A-game, and up the ante

Are you going to get better and then some more?
Do you have what it takes to enlighten and excel?
Can you learn to compete even when you cannot win?
Can you show the world what that means?

For at the end of the day, what really matters is not what comes your way but how you respond to it
And that is what separates
The also-ran from the greats

WELCOME HOME

(May 2017)

I love these two rejuvenating and patriotic words by the immigration officer at the airport. *Welcome home* is Mozart to my ears after a long flight back.

This time around, things may just be a little different as we return home from Hajj, the pilgrimage to Mecca, which is mandatory for all able Muslims once in their lifetime. This year it falls at the end of August, and my wife and I are planning on going.

The news is that since the Trump administration has taken over, there is extreme vetting of Muslims, among them many well-settled everyday Muslim American citizens. This process typically takes several hours, after an already long international flight.

As we are going through the planning stages for Hajj, the question in my mind is the following. We arrive at the JFK around noon on September 6th. Should we plan on getting home that night with a connecting flight or anticipate extreme vetting and several hours of delay and thus plan on staying another day in New York?

That I am in America for the last 25 years, a physician with a busy practice, having jumped through all the hoops of immigration and being vetted several times in the process. That I am part and parcel of the mainstream American fabric and that I am an American citizen. Nothing seemingly matters.

For I am a Muslim, and my name is Arif Ahmad.

An optimist at heart, I believe, these testing times would eventually pass. However, I would conclude by saying that this dangerous precedent of creating layers of citizenship is unconstitutional and never the way to make America great or safe again. If anything, this hits us hard at the very core of "We the People."

Ballieve me, as President Trump would say.

US MUSLIMS

(December 2015)

This is our circus, our monkeys.
The question begs how to best respond to all this.
Blame everyone else to the hilt for our ills.
Stay in our shell, shocked, shy, never to step out, never to mix.
Keep our eyes closed and pretend all is kosher.
Or wait for some other divine miracle.
Where each of us is a brand ambassador, I believe for a Muslim today, just showing up is not enough.
This is the time to step it up without apologies or excuses.
With smiling eyes and heads held high, at work or play, crawl if we have to go that extra mile.
To reach out, help out, love, impress.
Create some magic, make some good news, lay ourselves out to excel and embrace.
Step out from behind those walls.
Leave our surrounds a better place.

TRUMP'S RED HOT MIDDLE AMERICA AND HERE IS WHY

(November 2018)

I recently posted my archery buck picture and a complimentary poem on Facebook.

There were negative comments on my post aplenty. Here are some examples. Senseless, barbaric, cruel, deer meat is not palatable, killing the poor animals for pleasure, posting pictures of their dead bodies as trophies, have mercy, enjoy the moment of killing an animal soul for pleasure, and displaying it with pride, fishing is equally bad, saves lives during the day and takes lives during the night. The best of all compared the picture to putting foot over the face of the dead body of the enemy and getting it published.

Hunting for me is a small part of a much larger picture of connecting with nature. I grew up hunting with my family. I live, work and play in middle America. For a lot of middle America, hunting is a way of life. That is what they live, eat, celebrate, share and enjoy. The very same middle America who felt marginalized, and we all heard them loud and clear in 2016. I have friends, colleagues, neighbors, and patients from this middle America, and they are some of the best people I know. Many of them following along must have read these negative comments too.

Now many in America today complain about intolerance at the hands of this middle America. I want to show you all the flip side of this intolerance. Many in middle America live by hunting. Now read the above negative comments in light of reflecting on their way of life.

A Piece of Me

Please try and understand the Trump phenomenon. Being marginalized, criticized, judged poorly, and looked down upon for an extended period of time and thus.

We feel bad when intolerance comes our way but do we care for others when we dish it out? Tolerance, acceptance, coexistence, and love are always a two-way street, my dear all.

I hope we can all accept each other without prejudice and judgment, in spite of and embracing our differences. Amen.

TO APPNA

(June 2015, Association of Physicians of
Pakistani Descent of North America)

I leaned back in my chair and watched
The exuding happiness, the fanfare, the party galore
As my thoughts drifted away to the decades before
To our humble background, our ordinary beginnings
The starry-eyed wannabes
Willing to walk the tough miles, take the long road
We now stand arrived, the American dream realized
And realized every bit of good this great melting pot had on offer and wanting to share

As we shed our baggage, our insecurities and grew comfortable
We went ahead and put our best foot forward
Today we remain humble, grateful, and honored
As proud Pakistani Americans
Leaders, advocates, humanitarians, teachers, researchers, mentors, clinicians
All worthy, some in our own ways, in our own worlds
Yet it is as we come together that we become
This special fraternity, that distinctive someone

Let the magic continue as we rise higher
Soaring in the wings of each other
And back to the celebrations
Surrounded by friends
Happy to the point of being delirious
Feeding off each other's success

A Piece of Me

To our unity, our achievements
To that long road taken
To our time, to our era
We are the Association of Physicians of Pakistani Descent of North America

TIP OF THE ICEBERG

(November 2014)

Arriving on these shores a little later
I am some different
My culture, my sense of humor, my value set
Can you appreciate this, accept this?
That I have an accent
That I am dark and brown and from a distant planet
Can you respect me for who I am?
What I bring to the table
As an equal
No better, not worse
Stop being nervous
Call me Arif

Trust me as if I was blond and blue-eyed
Treat me as if I was white

Isn't this why we are who we are?
The United States worthy of this pale blue dot

THOSE MILE-LONG CHEVROLETS

(December 2014,
and I thought we were divided then)

The kid I was growing up loved watching the stars, and this one in particular which stood out bright
Ah, those mile-long Chevrolets, that postcard of New York City by night
This place they said where dreams come true
I would close my eyes, pretend and reach out to

Reach out I did, call it home
The season was "country before self"
The year was "give it your all"
And now some fulfilled dreams later
I hesitate, I ponder

This then those these the times have changed
Now in the age of self-siege and standoff
Of partisan jousting and deadlock
Taking some serious heat, getting beat, my dreams, and my star
Turning into sand
I am frantically trying holding on to, in my clenched hand

THINK IT OVER ANY WHICH WAY

(March 2015, as we stay fighting)

All of us the intense enemies of today
Till the moment that hand of nature strikes
Something of the proportions which took the dinosaurs away
Remember the civilizations which this earth now hides
And in the ensuing mayhem
What happens to our ongoing fights?
Would we stay fighting or stop?
Help only our own or just about anyone?
Think it over any which way
Why wait for a catastrophe to unite us, I say

THE WORKOUT

(June 2013)

For the love of what I do
For the cardiologist in me
To practice what I preach
To inspire myself and to inspire you
I workout

When I feel low, down, and knocked out
To fight my inner demons and negative vibes
To handle stress better
To moan, groan, express myself and vent my frustrations
For the high, I get after
I workout

To pursue my passions, my goals, my aspirations
To feed my pride and boost my confidence
To look and feel my best
To be a responsible citizen
To appreciate and be thankful that I can
I workout

For the love of eating
For my daily fix, my daily high
To protect against the ravages of time and disease
To be able to make this pitch to you
I workout

Arif Ahmad

To caress my aching body and soothe my tired mind
To cleanse my soul and rejuvenate my spirits and spirituality
Some days intense, some days just easy, some days dragging myself
I workout

And one day die I will, die I shall but before my time is up to live every day to its fullest
I workout

JULY 2020

The United States Declaration of Independence still reads,

To prove this, let Facts be submitted to a candid world.

He has refused his Assent to Laws, the most wholesome and necessary for the public good.

He has endeavoured to prevent the population of these States; for that purpose obstructing the Laws for Naturalization of Foreigners; refusing to pass others to encourage their migrations hither, and raising the conditions of new Appropriations of Lands.

He has obstructed the Administration of Justice, by refusing his Assent to Laws for establishing Judiciary powers.

He has made Judges dependent on his Will alone, for the tenure of their offices, and the amount and payment of their salaries.

He has combined with others to subject us to a jurisdiction foreign to our constitution, and unacknowledged by our laws; giving his Assent to their Acts of pretended Legislation.

For cutting off our Trade with all parts of the world.

For taking away our Charters, abolishing our most valuable Laws, and altering fundamentally the Forms of our Governments.

A Prince whose character is thus marked by every act which may define a Tyrant, is unfit to be the ruler of a free people.

THE RESET

(June 2015)

I retraced my steps and checked every nook and corner, every which where way except for the ocean floor. It was gone for sure. My pictures, my connection to the internet and the rest of the world, everything. I had lost my cell phone. I felt devastated, and my mood went from a high high to a low low.

I was out in the middle of nowhere on day three of this Alaskan hunting and fishing adventure. Constantly shuffling between land and water, I had it in my shirt pocket and never saw it drop or heard a sound. I was on a logging trail when I realized it was missing. The last picture on it was the beautiful red snapper I had caught about thirty minutes ago. It felt as if my life had been sucked out of me. I felt awful, just plain and simple.

I tried some psychotherapy, telling myself that this is not the worst which could have happened. Still out in the boonies, having lost my pictures and not being able to get on the internet using the camp Wi-Fi was a bit too much and all too soon to handle.

And what about the daily dose of Facebook?

It rubbed in even more that out in the Alaskan wild, I had no chance to replace it for the next several days. With whales, bears, and bald eagles against the magnificent backdrop, I was already missing my next selfie. I was withdrawing and clearly showing signs of a cell phone junkie.

Day two was perhaps a little better, and day three even more so. My friends with me picked up the slack. Thank you, Dave, Steve, Chris, and Kyle.

And then I surprised myself. By day five and six, I started liking it.

In some ways coming off this cell phone addiction, I felt detoxified, cleansed, and liberated.

I felt assured that I controlled my cell phone and not vice versa. It reminded me of the days gone by when there were none. Instead of taking endless pictures, it made me absorb and appreciate the scenery. It forced me not to check the news and email for the umpteenth time each day and not be consumed by the internet.

And thanks are due to my friend, Google, who had my back and had saved most of my pictures and contacts.

Now back home, I am still riding this wave of empowerment, of control, and this time around, purposely delaying getting the new phone. Ultimately, I would have to get one, though the Alaskan wilderness taught me a valuable lesson. In more than one way, it tested my body, my mind, my spirit.

It gave me a welcome reset.

EARLY IN THE PANDEMIC

(April 2020)

the hunter's instinct is to hunt it down
the scientist to contain it till a cure is found
the physician stays up knowing worse is around
Dear God, if You are there
What is Your point here?

THE GIRL OF MY DREAMS

(July 2014)

The year was 1988. I had just finished medical school and was into the first few weeks of residency at a government hospital in Lahore, Pakistan.

It was an afternoon. As luck would have it, I was covering some doctors and, in effect, by myself in the ward. These were the days before the cell phones and beepers. Usually, a landline phone, if working, or person to person contact, was the way to communicate.

I remember feeling good, confident, in control, and why not? I was a physician now, a complete package, the real deal, and in charge of that moment, or so I thought. If only I knew what was coming.

A ward boy came to the doctor's office to summon me with some urgency. There was something terribly wrong; I could tell from his looks. In the corridor outside was a small girl, no more than 5 or 6 years old, in the lap of her mother. The girl appeared listless and was crying but in a strange and weak voice. The mother had no clue what had happened. I was soon to realize that neither did I.

It all happened very fast, in a few minutes, minutes which felt like an eternity. As I was frantically trying to come up with some possibilities or solutions, the other staff went around looking for more senior, more experienced doctors. I have to say that out in a corridor some distance from the emergency room, in a race against time, I was hoping against hope that this situation would fix itself.

The girl became quieter and lethargic by the minute. A small crowd of passersby had formed, and I could feel the weight of their expectations. I tried listening to her breath sounds, in this by now, a noisy and panicky situation, and could not tell. The bookish strength of my diagnosis and management had long vanished, and I felt just as helpless, if not more than this little girl in front of me.

Her pulse was barely palpable. That I did a Heimlich thinking of a foreign body actually happened or is just a figment of my imagination, I am not sure. In any case, the girl slowed down further and finally died right in front of my eyes, still in her mother's lap. That was the end of it for her and a rude awakening for me. Her cause of death could not be ascertained. It was the first person I ever saw dying, a child and on my watch.

This girl, I do not have a name for, lives on, in my mind, my soul, and now my writing.
The question I beg to ask all our modern-day killers is.
What is in your psyche, and how do you live with it?

THE AMERICAN GUN LAW PARADOX

(March 2018)

As I see our youth spearheading the current national Gun Law Movement and debate, I wonder.

Typically, the young are more adventurous and risk-takers, and their parents and elders more cautious and risk-averse. Typically, the elders would do anything and everything in their power to try and decrease any real or perceived risk for their children and more acutely so if the young ones ask for such help.

What we are witnessing in America may be the exact opposite of this.

The support for gun control is highest among 18 to 29-year-olds and lowest among 50 to 64 and 65 plus age groups, a study by the Pew Research Center suggests.

It appears that the American youth are trying to rein in the risk to their lives and living, and it is the American elders, and especially the ones who matter the most in the Congress, who are slow to react.

It seems that our youth are asking for less of guns, and their elders are insisting that they keep more.

TAKE A KNEE

(October 2017)

Rapturous applause following, "Fire that SOB."
This for taking a knee.
Seriously?

Since when is kneeling considered disrespectful. I would have understood if it was something obnoxious or obscene, but kneeling?

I would argue that to take a knee to the Anthem and the Flag and to allow that to happen is one of the most American things to do. Here is why.

REST OF THE WORLD
At many places on this planet, protest and dissent are not acceptable. People are punished, jailed, and killed for doing the same. We as Americans fight such practices ideologically by setting and emphasizing our example of allowing and tolerating peaceful protest. Our Military fights wars to try and protect our way of life so we can do just that. To be able to take a knee is holding on to everything which our Flag stands for and our Military defends.

OUR BIRTH
The United States of America was born out of discontent, dismay, and revolt against, among other things, not having a voice. Taking a knee is a voice that needs to be heard.

OUR CONSTITUTION
The supreme document of the Land, our Constitution guarantees these freedoms, expressions, and assembly. The Flag, the Anthem, the Military are

all symbols, extensions, and guardians of these rights, these liberties, and our Constitution.

ONLY IN AMERICA

We Americans are unique. Doing things differently is ingrained in our DNA. We exercise and express our freedoms unabashedly and boldly. Taking a knee is an unusual way of protesting. To allow such protest is American. To discuss why and bring positive change, as a result even more so. It is this last step, which for us usually takes the longest. The real discussion here can be about justice and equality, not just on paper but in reality.

THE RIGHT THING TO DO

To disagree with the idea is all right, to disallow it is not. To have a discourse is okay, to abuse and punish is not. Almost always, sooner or later, America comes around to do the right thing. We have to ask our better selves.
What is the right thing to do here?

STRUGGLE

(August 2015)

Annoyed at him, issues with her
Never content for one reason or the other
Often projecting my own shortcomings, my own failures
And them temptations, temptations, temptations
I seem to love being my own biggest struggle

STATE OF PAKISTAN

(December 2014)

Who are you really, they ask me?
I am not sure, maybe a free spirit, a confused nobody?
Born a Muslim Sunni, half Arain, half Pathan, a Punjabi
This now is not my real identity
Today I am a terrorized Hindu, a lynched Christian, a torched Shia, a scared Ahmadi
Today I am every persecuted Pathan, Baloch, Muhajir, and Sindhi
I was there with the children of Peshawar on that school floor
I am the collateral damage of all war
I am in all political spheres
And I am not a terrorist, for a terrorist, with a terrorist and shall never be
I am a Pakistani
But more than that
I belong to this universal family
A fraternity called humanity

REALITY CHECK

(June 2019, APPNA is the Association
of Physicians of Pakistani Descent of North America)

Got the reconciliation news in APPNA again for the umpteenth time
Kudos to all involved, but wait a second, not so fast
I am not clapping, not just yet
Before we start giving each other a pat on the back
Allow me to read out our report card

Elections or no elections, we play politics with or without a reason
We fight in print, in person, at all levels, for all positions
Not just the BOT and EC, chapters and alumni
We even politicize, pressurize, twist arms for committees
And why not for we are this indispensable gift from God
We hold the time, we own the place
APPNA should feel indebted, keep delivering us its all

Our history tells me this truce is temporary
Soon we shall be back to our old ways
Slapping hard at our ever-shrinking face
The daggers we hold behind our backs
Our battle lines are permanent, our politics is revenge
Who runs this hate machine?
Where lies the head of this snake?
Slaves of our bitter history, we cannot break free
Our better work is optional, our fights mandatory
Forget we don't, forgive we never
Animus amongst us is forever

A Piece of Me

Our conundrum always had a solution
Clear and present in our constitution
That line in the sand called,
Accept the vote by the supreme authority
Respect the will of the General Body
Become an honest democracy

AS AN AMERICAN MUSLIM

(August 2016, I had emailed this writing
to the White House. President Obama's reply follows)

I can keep my eyes closed and report that all is hunky-dory, that all is well just because nothing untoward has happened to me yet.
Or I can be honest.
The war has come home and in a bad way, for such is the nature of this beast, and the price is being asked of and paid by those having nothing to do with it.

As it happens in such scenarios, the scale of the problem gets exaggerated several times over as in the number of deaths in America from terrorism is still a tiny fraction of those from gun violence.
With all due respect, would the dead have known or cared for the difference? Victims remain victims, and why are we choosing between them?

Whichever way I slice it, this is not just a rhetoric anymore. The American Muslims are taking some serious heat and are a growing target.
Many are between a rock and a hard place, for their native countries are torn and in a state of perpetual conflict.
From being the low-hanging fruit in the war zones of the East to facing prejudice in the West, we now make that perfect sandwich.

On tenterhooks, walking on eggshells, never thought it would come to this, not here in the US.
Listening to the commentary, I wonder if we are going to be played with or eaten, for it'll take the best of the American values and the law of the land to protect us.

A Piece of Me

Tough it out we shall, and keep our fingers crossed and hope against hope, things settle down, cool off.
P for Patience, P for Positive, P for Peace, one letter and three words, still make for an incomplete sentence.
I am asking you for a way to come out better and stronger through this.

PRESIDENT OBAMA'S REPLY

(September 7, 2016)

THE WHITE HOUSE
WASHINGTON

Thank you for writing. When any religious group is targeted, we all have a responsibility to speak up. As Americans, we must stay true to our core values, and that includes freedom of religion for all faiths. Though it may sometimes seem like the angriest and loudest voices are controlling our national discourse, I want you to know that I believe in the power of our kindest and most thoughtful voices to build a more welcoming and inclusive society, and in the power of our laws to protect the rights of all people. The same Amendment that gives our country's citizens the right to speak freely also gives people of different backgrounds and religions the ability to practice their faith how they choose—and Muslims were among those our Founders had in mind when they wrote it.

Muslim Americans have played an important role in shaping our Nation's character since our beginning—serving as community leaders who guide us forward, athletes and artists who inspire us, entrepreneurs who boost our economy, and men and women in uniform who give of themselves so we may live in peace and security. The contributions of Muslim Americans have helped write a strong, resilient American narrative, and we will not stop defending the right of all our people to live safely and with dignity—no matter who they are, where they come from, or what religion they practice.

Again, thank you for writing. Please know your message will remain on my mind.

Sincerely,
Barack Obama

PREZ O

(February 2016, to President Obama)

My Dear Prez O
Congrats on your last year in office
You have done right, some more than the others
And you have faltered, recovered
Kind at heart, and you have tried
As we saw your hair turn white
Though, there is something
The big leaders lead
The great ones unite
Somehow they rise above the strife
So, Prez O, can you try even harder and bring us together, please
For our country, this world, your very own legacy

PLEASE

(October 2017,
after the Las Vegas shooting)

Recently a patient of mine, a chronic heavy smoker, quit smoking. He says, "Doc in the after-visit summary it said, "Please quit smoking" and no one had ever asked me "Please" before."
I will try this charm and see if I can get lucky again, realizing that this one is a rather stiff ask.

I find myself somewhere between gloomy and more gloomy since the Vegas raining bullets massacre. Gloomy because I know the next one will happen and then another and another. We the people, seem unable to help ourselves. The next place in America, this will happen, and the number of casualties is as if playing a game of darts, blindfolded, or pulling out a lottery slip from a bucket full of all our names and towns in it.

Here are some statistics on mass shootings defined as four or more victims, excluding the shooter. America leads the rest of the World hands down and averages almost one mass shooting a day. Yes, nine out of ten days on average. Semi-automatic firearms with high capacity magazines are the weapons of choice. More than half of the shooters are white males. Terrorists have killed only a fraction of these but make the most hoopla in the news.

You think this will never happen to you. Well, check with the survivors of Vegas and Orlando. Each time something like this happens, everyone hopes that the perpetrator is not one of them. Terrorist is the buzzword if a Muslim does it. Evil is the word used if it is someone else.

The numbers keep going up, the idea of killing as many in as little time possible, as in a weird and ugly competition. Typically the hunting rifles and shotguns shoot up to four shells. That is all one needs for fair game. Revolvers hold six rounds. Those were the good old days.

Enter semi-automatic weapons with large-capacity magazines. A bolt action hunting rifle needs to be actioned after firing each round. A semi-automatic weapon, in contrast, can keep shooting one at a time till there are bullets in the magazine, which may be dozens. A fully automatic rifle fires in continuous rapid bursts, the kind of sounds heard in Vegas.

It turns out that a semi-automatic rifle can be turned into a fully automatic one rather easily and illegally with the addition of a bump stock. Even the NRA now wants these bump stocks regulated. Try regulating the semi-automatic weapons themselves, and you are out of luck. That ain't happening, and there is nothing we can do about it except keep dying and keep on trying.

Three countries have successfully regulated against these mass killings. The United Kingdom after the tragedy of Dunblane, Australia after that of Port Arthur and Germany after the incident in Winnenden. Stricter gun laws, ban of rapid-fire weapons, and Government buyback were some of the things that were done.

The argument to be armed to the teeth to protect against bad elements can mean that if tomorrow crooks show up with rocket launchers, we may also start selling them at Cabela's. The argument that the bad actors will get them anyway can mean that we can make freely available crack cocaine, heroin, and other drugs. The argument that an armed vigilante is the best remedy to prevent such an attack means that we would have to arm a lot more people for all places at all times.

Think it over for a second. These tactical, combat, large magazine guns are doing precisely what they are meant to do and are the weapons of choice for mass murderers, for they are readily and freely available. Walmart made the call and stopped selling semi-automatic weapons as an example of American corporate conscience. What about others?

The serial killers of the past had to work for their killings. Today it is far too easy. Only so many people can be killed with a knife, a bolt action rifle, or a revolver. It is these rapid-fire weapons with magazines holding dozens of bullets that have changed the landscape. The more the eggs, the bigger is the omelet, the more the rounds fired rapidly, the bigger is the carnage. How many more need to die before we can influence change?

The technology would only keep getting better with more sophisticated weaponry with more mass killing capability. We went to a full war in Iraq to protect its people and neighbors from weapons of mass destruction and indiscriminate killing. Does raining bullets, 59 dead, over 500 injured qualify for mass destruction? Does a mass shooting almost every day in America feel like a war zone? This has to be a curse, for seemingly, we cannot do much about this problem.

I am a hunter. I own strings and arrows and guns myself. I have friends who are the same, and we are all very passionate about our rights and the second amendment. So I am going to say it differently.

My dear gun-loving Americans, this is in our hands, if we can come together as one and at the very least do away with the semi-automatic weapons. Please.
If nothing else for the sake of our children.

PINK

(March 2017)

People pitched against People,
for the right of passage
Action and reaction,
equal and opposite
My two hands,
left and right,
fight
Turn it over,
to the Women
On a journey between a male chauvinist and a feminist
Pink it
Clap with one hand and with the other erase legacy
I to mine and you play to your gallery
Decency
What decency?
Abstract honesty
Pink is the new me
Not white, black, brown, yellow
There is simply one
Of love, friendship, kindness
The shade we are born in
Pink is us

PARIS, JANUARY 7th, 2015

(Charlie Hebdo incident.
This writing was published online by the CNN)

Last day in France, our wedding anniversary, on a visit to that one Louvre and the Eiffel Tower.

It turns grim about midday with news of the Charlie massacre.

A friend then urged me,
"Arif, you are a Muslim, and here is an opportunity."
"Write something."
And I am thinking,
Get in the middle of this mess, are you kidding?

For how should I ask the civilized world if freedom of speech means compulsive insulting of a religion, and where its prophet's imagery is forbidden, repeatedly making his funny caricatures?

And how am I conveying it to the Muslims that the "Law of Sarcasm" states that the more sensitive one is about something, the more likely it will keep hitting them in the face?

How am I going to say that maybe a vacuum exists for lack of a more sophisticated response by a Muslim scholar?

And how in the world can I tell the Muslim fundamentalists that reactionary killing is negative publicity, a self-defeating prophecy, the exact opposite of Allah ho Akbar?

So I am staying out of this as that I believe is better.

PAKISTAN ZINDABAD
(LONG LIVE PAKISTAN)

(November 2013)

The first part of this story is how it was narrated to me by my father. The year was 1947. India Pakistan partition had just taken place, and my father, who was the eldest of the siblings in the family, had a task at hand. In the midst of senseless and rampant killing on both sides of the border targeting one of the biggest human migrations in history, he had to move his family from Jullundur India to Lahore, Pakistan, and to do it safely. The family consisted of his aging and sick parents and younger siblings.

A large truck was acquired to accomplish this feat. The family, with all their worldly possessions, were loaded up. Father stood on a high platform watching guard with a gun in his hand. He placed the gun strategically with the barrel emerging from under a raincoat and clearly visible as a deterrent.

On the way to Lahore, they passed violent mobs and insane scenes of blood and gory, which I would rather take a pass on describing. Their truck with father at a watch with his gun at ready was understandably left alone to arrive safely in Lahore and for me to be able to write about this decades later.

I witnessed the second part of this story. I was there. It was some year in the 1980s. As a young man and pursuing my family's passion, I was big into hunting. At any given opportunity, and especially the weekends, our party of friends and family would venture out in several different areas around Lahore to enjoy the outdoors and the sport.

This was a night hunt for wild boars around the BRB canals near Lahore, Pakistan. We were in an open Willys Jeep. An open Jeep means that the soft top cover has been removed, and the front screen is laid down on the bonnet. This gives the hunters easy access to see and hunt game.

It had to be a fall evening, as I remember feeling a little chilly. We were on the mud road by the canal, heading deeper into the woods. The canal was to our right, and the open crop fields with interspersed patches of tall brown grass to our left. We were probably 6-8 people that night and with a variety of weapons, including shotguns, rifles, and pistols, and ready for action. I sat in one of the rear seats behind the driver.

We were cruising at a slow speed, approximately 15 mph. One person in the back was standing and shining a spotlight, looking for game. From the corner of my eye, I remember seeing a faint figure of a man in khaki shalwar kameez, the traditional Pakistani dress, along the side of the road some hundred yards upfront. This man then jumped right in front of us onto the mud road and started walking towards the jeep. We could see him clearly in our lights while he had to be blinded looking into them. As we slowed down, the man brought up his hands, shouldering his rifle and aiming straight at us. He then yelled in a loud and clear voice, "Halt."

We did stop. The standoff continued for a few tense moments. With a crisp, confident and clear voice, the man asked who we were. My uncle in the front seat replied with our identity and purpose. After what felt like an eternity, the man dropped his arms and lowered his weapon. He then walked up to the jeep and, by now comfortable with our identity, introduced himself as an on-duty Ranger, a paramilitary force in Pakistan, on his regular nightly patrol.

Fast forward to 2013. I was in Pakistan for a family wedding. One of my class fellows and a good friend is the head of the department of cardiac surgery at a local government teaching hospital. He invited me to come and spend some time in their department over a couple of days, and I gladly obliged. It was an eye-opener. They are doing off-pump, complete arterial graft cardiac bypass surgeries. In plain English, it means the state-of-the-art work.

These three stories are decades apart and span the life of Pakistan. What is the common link and my point in bringing them up?

The cardiac surgery team is producing state-of-the-art work with meager resources, the bare minimum, available to them.

All that Ranger's Jawan had on him for a weapon that night was a stick, which he simulated as a gun to perform his duty in challenging and checking on a jeep load of hunters with a variety of loaded weapons.

Father had no gun on him for that move during the partition. He crossed the killing fields and delivered his family safely with the metal end of a folded umbrella drawn out of a raincoat and feigning as a rifle.

What all these people have in common is the minimum of resources, but the abundance of ingenuity, self-belief, and confidence, and the will to take on the world against all odds. All these people are true patriots and my heroes, and I know there are many more like them.

It has to be Pakistan Zindabad all the way.

PAIN

(July 2018)

I am feeling numb.
Numb what?

To say something.
Say what?

To write something.
Write what?

To plead with you.
Plead what?

That we are all human.
What?

OPTIMISM ON THE ROPES

(April 2013)

I live in the realm of hurt, in the kingdom of pain.

The religion of peace and our age held hostage by a handful of radicals. The savage and the hidden few, killing left, right, and center, innocents and bystanders, women and children and wreaking havoc with their twisted ideology and a Jihad gone astray.

Haqooq-ul-Ibad who cares, Sharia and Quran misinterpreted, defied.

The Muslim scholars, the political powers, divided, scared, dumbfounded, and quiet, watching from the sidelines, feeling safe and protected, their heads in the sand.

Our youth, our poor youth, between a rock and a hard place, confused, disillusioned, discouraged, and turning away.

More than anyone else, Muslims killing Muslims, a shameful statistic, not easy to explain, not easy to defend.

These barbaric acts, justified as revenge, retaliation, without remorse and mercy and not realizing that:

Two wrongs never make a right.

"Hope for peace" are three words, as are "Not in sight."

Optimism on the ropes.

I live in the realm of hurt, in the kingdom of pain.

ONE EARTH, ONE SPECIES

(August 2017)

A wise man once said,
though in a different context,
action and reaction,
are equal and opposite.

A not as wise man now says,
abuse generates more abuse,
hate begets more hate.
As species, we are bent upon self-eradication.
Little realizing that we are in this together.

I work to conserve this land, to preserve human life.
What is it you do for existence?

ONE AND ONE

(February 2019)

Can our one and one equal eleven?
pause
disbelief
laughter

Seven?
pause
all right
I get it

Can our one and one equal two?

ON OUR VERY OWN

(May 2014, Pakistan. A pregnant woman was stoned to death in the tradition of honor killing, and a doctor was murdered for being a religious minority.)

I feel tired and sleepy
Playing out our obituary
For getting stoned is this woman
Pregnant
Waiting to be forgotten
Like the rest of us
Who died that day with her
She is hemorrhaging
I am standing still in a silent crowd
Watching

Playing the musical chairs of death
We go around in circles
Cutting our own feet
Slitting our own throats
Stabbing each other in the back
That color on me, that red
Is it mine or someone else's blood

Who is next up for sacrifice?
The next Doctor Mehdi Ali
You or me
If death had a wish
We can all perish

A Piece of Me

To give future a chance
May be

To all those who want to bring us, people, down
Let it be known
Just back off
Leave us alone
For we shall finish ourselves
On our very own

OF I AND ME

(April 2014)

My will and want, my drive, and the choice between right and wrong
I battle myself in the same old battleground
Here I can walk the clouds and conquer the world
Or fall from grace with a loud thud
Here I can be my own best friend
Or stay on as my worse enemy yet

Here I can work to improve on my story
Here I can fly, aim high, reach for glory
Take a leap or do it a step at a time
Though there is that one small matter
Left for me to master
Of I and Me
To let go of my fears
Take charge of my mind
Assume control of my being

NEWS

(May 2016)

News of gloom
That of the impending doom
Negative news and then some
That lump in the throat
Reporting on the ugly, broadcasting the terrible
Over and over
A disproportionately pessimistic view of this world
Dampening of the good, exaggerating the bad
Keeping us on the hook and edge
Calling one disaster after another
Ignoring most of which is better
And our misery addicted minds
(Misery often that of the others)
Keep buying into this sick sensationalism
A frustrating experience it is
Most of what we get as News
Whatever sells and is good for business
I guess

NO NEED FOR ELECTION REFORMS IN APPNA

(June 2018, Satire)

Na yar Gumrah, don't you say the!

Elections are fun so, please don't ruin them, with candidates swooning around the voters, their wallets leaking tens of thousands of dollars, the gossiping, the backbiting, the hardcore politicking.

Yes, the elections bring out the worst amongst us, but who is keeping logs, and who really cares. Imagine the opportunities, the canvassing, when life and death hang in the balance, the arm twisting, the joy of a few over the agony of many, and of course the infighting which later spills outside.

We get to relish every bit of it and precisely why the circus stays at where it is.

So my dear, let the crazy, gut-wrenching election cycles be, for, under the skin of a 501 (c), APPNA might be a political heavyweight wannabe.

Now contrast all this to the listless, email or paper ballot, no noise elections at our hospitals and medical societies, where often we do not have a face to a name; blah that to our exciting game.

Fake or real, ire or satire, before I seek change, is the voter in me willing to change its desire?

NATION OF SIMILAR ONLY

(March 2018, facing
racism at home in the USA)

Recently a piece of news caught my eye, and for a reason when the Interior Secretary Ryan Zinke was quoted by several for his repeated comments against workplace diversity, something which he denies.

In any case, this made me realize and now write about my own experience from not so far back when two men who I have known for a long time said to me that they believe similar people should live together as a nation and repeated that line to make sure I heard and understood it.

To give all this a little more meaning, these two are educated white male Christians, while the last I checked, yours truly, still remains a brown Muslim. The comment was out of the blue and out of context with anything relevant we were discussing at that time, and it caught me by surprise.

Even though I realize that the comment was meant for me being different, at that time, I just ignored it.

Now I guess it implied that similar looking people should live together as a nation, or it could have been the same religion, or both, I cannot be certain as I never sought clarification. The immigration status could not have been a factor as one of the two is an immigrant, just like me.

With the current wave of nationalism, let us assume for a moment that similar people should live together as a nation then here are just a few interesting situations I can think of, and I am sure there are many more where the boundaries based on race, color, and religion get blurred.

There are a lot of white Muslims with light eyes. Do they belong with the Muslims or with the whites?

Would the darker shades of Christians live with their color or with white Christians?

What about the Atheists?

How about the native Americans, the original residents? Would they stay or look for a different universe?

Who gets to decide all of this?

THE INSPIRATION THAT IS AN AMERICAN PRESIDENT

(December 2018, published by the AP)

Youth all over the globe look up to the American President. Years ago, growing up in Pakistan, I was one such youth.

How can they be so gracious to their opponents, the ease with which they put the country before self, their better ideals translating the larger World issues, their standing up in the face of tyranny, genocide, and brutal dictators, their grace, poise, and reflection, their push for excellence and always for a better tomorrow, the list goes on and on.

Still, no one living person or position on the planet is more influential than that of the American President and especially for the younger generations and thereby shaping the future of this world in more ways than we all realize.

Some things of late have distorted this image, though.

Clinton's cigars, a personal failing, took some away from an otherwise fine stint and reminded me that Presidents are, after all, human.

The reverberations of W's bad Intel War are still being felt today, though George W. Bush was a decent person, and I am not sure if any other President would have reacted differently to the same Intel.

However, the damage being done to the Office of the American Presidency and American repute at large by Trump et al. is in a league of its own. How much of this damage is salvageable once America and the World are done with Trump is held by the morrow.

The 24/7 news with analysis and over-analysis may be helping Trump to distract by promptly spreading the banana peels and continuing to muddy the waters.

As the World awaits good and decent people to lead America again, may long live the seat of the American Presidency and through it our value system of a Leader Nation through example, inspiration, and doing the right thing with or against the odds.

OUR BELOVED APPNA

(January 2019, APPNA is the Association of Physicians of Pakistani descent of North America. This self-critique should not take away from loads of good APPNA does. It is inspired by this popular line in our communications.)

our beloved appna
aren't you glad
we are
a mere
three thousand
for we have repeatedly
slapped you, stabbed you
incited mutiny
broken your discipline
dispensed confusion
encouraged alternate groups
for chaos and rebellion
threatened our fellow members
with consequences
dealt in harassment
of all sorts
dragged you in the courts
enjoyed and participated
to the hilt
in perpetual conflicts
championed democracy
dismissing majority
never sorry

Arif Ahmad

always eager
for only we can
take you higher
make you better
you remain
our beloved Appna
now and forever

MY JESUS MOMENT

(May 2020)

A routine plays out at my place of work year after year. I call it my Jesus moment.

Every year I fast during Ramadan. For those not sure, this is a Muslim tradition of no eating or drinking from pre-dawn to sunset for a month straight. It is a spiritual and physical cleansing and reckoning of sorts.

Kathy, a colleague of mine, is an excellent pastry chef, a bakester par excellence. That she is Christian and married to a pastor adds a little more oomph to this storyline.

For years now, I would do the fasting, and Kathy would bake a cake and other confectionery for the department to celebrate the end of Ramadan.

I bear the brunt for the good of many—my Jesus moment. We get a laugh out of it.

Even more, in the World of today, I derive hope out of this.

MY BROTHER

(March 2018)

Gun violence hits me close to home.

I once had a brother, a younger brother, Abid. He owned a less than perfect life in more than one way. The place was Lahore, Pakistan; the decade was the 1980s, mother had cancer, the struggle, the suffering, her death, and Abid suffered with her, perhaps more than her. She passed on, and his struggles piled on.

We all tried to help, we made our own mistakes in the process, we all failed. We explored multiple venues, including psychiatric help and treatment for depression. Nothing worked. Abid succumbed to a self-inflicted gunshot wound. Accident or suicide, we will never know. Mental issues or not, I do not know. What I know is that only one person was hurt on that ill-fated night and no one else.

In retrospect, he was probably depressed in a time when mental illness of any kind was considered taboo, and there were hardly any psychiatrists available. He ended up seeing a General Physician, and the prescribed medicines only made him more groggy and did not help.

That mental health is getting blamed for American mass shootings is not corroborated by the available data or by the experts in the field. The available data may even be to the contrary.

As a physician, I live my life in an evidence-based world. I will quote two examples of why research is essential.

CAST was a landmark trial looking to suppress extra heartbeats after a heart attack with certain antiarrhythmic drugs. The extra beats did decrease, but the death rate in the treated group increased significantly.

More recently, the drugs to raise the good cholesterol though good, in theory, either showed no clinical benefit or actual harm.

The bottom line, unless backed by quality research, it remains a hypothesis.

In the United States, a country on top of the World with its R&D and evidence-based living, where is the research on gun violence?

Well, it is not allowed by a "Dickey Amendment" and financial arm-twisting of the CDC (Centers for Disease Control and Prevention) since 1996. Interestingly in his later years, Jay Dickey, the congressman from Arkansas, had changed his position and became a vocal and written proponent of research into American gun violence.

Jay Dickey and Mark Rosenberg of CDC, opponents, turned allies, co-wrote a famous Op-ed in The Washington Post in 2012 and said this,

"We were on opposite sides of the heated battle 16 years ago, but we are in strong agreement now that scientific research should be conducted into preventing firearm injuries and that ways to prevent firearm deaths can be found without encroaching on the rights of legitimate gun owners. The same evidence-based approach that is saving millions of lives from motor-vehicle crashes, as well as from smoking, cancer and HIV/AIDS, can help reduce the toll of deaths and injuries from gun violence."

So, who is responsible here? The mentally ill being blamed for the American gun violence scourge on a whim and without supporting evidence and research or the self-professed mentally sane rest of us who have chosen to block research on this issue and have repeatedly failed to implement measures to make a difference?

Who are the sane, and who are the ill?

MY APOLOGY

(April 2017)

Self before nation always.
Loud, pompous, jealous.
Living beyond my means.
Front-loaded with apathy.
No, not really.
I am a Pakistani.

Stolen wealth, now my money is to launder and hide.
Taxes, what taxes?
Constipated accountability.
Corrupt are the politicians only.
I pay my share diligently.
Maybe.
I am a Pakistani.

License to kill anyone, anywhere, based on blasphemy.
Intolerance is my specialty.
You are at fault, it's never me.
I have contacts, and I have money.
A culture of VIP, VVIP.
Never mind the fellow citizens, the country, the weak, the minority.
All that matters is my and me.
Fixing the ills is not my duty.
Others are corrupt from A to Z.
This is all a conspiracy.
I am a Pakistani.

A Piece of Me

Albeit for a worthy few,
there won't be a go-round,
or a merry.
Quit messing with me.
I am a Pakistani.
My apology.

MUSIC OUT OF A PHYSICIAN'S KEYBOARD

(August 2015)

Noble profession check, recession-proof check, my love, passion and one of the few things I do well, check

I am and always will be a physician first till my last breath

But slowly, steadily, of late, things have changed

Once so eager to have my children become doctors to recently when they announced that is not what they would want to become, I actually felt relieved

The gloss coming off this profession is now clear and present but started slow and at multiple places all together

The misuse, overuse, abuse of available resources

The cost of litigation and its dreaded fear factor

Dwindling reimbursements to and fading away of private practices

And with wars and maiming taking precedence over preserving and improving life, it may be an issue with our priorities

As the regulations, paperwork, and oversight ballooned, the physicians ceded control of their destiny by choice and out of laziness, and the vacuum was filled by business people, administrators with whom they now share, at times, a love-hate relationship

Why?

Let's just call it the stress of walking this tightrope and feeding many a more mouth on this ever-shrinking pie

Healthcare of today is a nasty, cut-throat, do or die business

Stay in black and survive, develop a liking for red and perish

The margins for many hospitals are bare-bones, while those for the industry are in hundreds of millions

And the physicians of today are bossed around and at the mercy of many, left guessing, tentative, looking over their shoulders, waiting to be made an example of

And them ever contracting RVUs, compensated for initially by working longer and doing more

Though not anymore, with so much else competing for the physician's time, last checked, the hours in a day were still only twenty-four

Today and with no disrespect intended, a plumber, an electrician, a car mechanic often charge more per hour than a doctor

Besides, there is no other profession I know which gets paid cents on the dollar

Try that with your internet or any other service provider or at a restaurant after dinner

And talk of loving it between a rock and a hard place for being a cardiologist is in itself a cardiac risk factor

With human lives at the receiving end, the ask is to keep doing more, of higher quality and for less

And with no end in sight for this squeeze yet, this is an awkward balancing act

Please do not take me wrong, for physicians in America are still at the cutting edge of medicine and better off than many others

And most of us are going to fade away and live it out as is, for this is how we know to pay our bills

But for the years which go into it, the studying, the training, the stress of never-ending exams and life in general, the expectations, the responsibility, the endless work hours, unless one loves it dearly, it just may not be worth it anymore

Except for all those sick yet beautiful and appreciative patients

That is when the years spent perfecting and practicing this art and science make perfect sense

"ME TOO" OF A DIFFERENT KIND

(February 2018, after yet
another mass shooting in the USA)

Another mass shooting tragedy in America. We are all too emotional right now; this is not the time to talk gun control is what we are told.

In a week or so, when the pain lessens for most of us, so does the passion for change, so why talk gun control then?

Weeks later, the last incident forgotten, wiped off our memories, greed in full control, gun control, what gun control?

So my dear fellow Americans, as you see, there is no good time to be talking gun control.

They also cite the constitution, which clearly states, "the right of the people to keep and bear semi-automatic turned automatic Arms with high capacity magazines, shall not be infringed."

For me, this remains an example of American Men messing up this issue beyond recognition. Even though the rest of the modern world has found its way around this problem with gun control laws, that is not our issue, we are repeatedly told.

Maybe, just maybe, the gathering American Women power can jump in to wade us all out of this mess.

Or the speed with which the communities and people affected by mass shootings are increasing, this may well turn into another "Me Too" movement.

So wait patiently, America, for all the powerful who can but are refusing to protect us from this scourge; wait patiently for enough of them and theirs to become part of this "Me Too," and that is precisely when we would have our gun control laws.

It is only a matter of time and statistics.

DEAR GOD
THE GRIEVANCE AND THE RESPONSE

(November 2013, inspired by
the genius of Dr. Allama Iqbal)

Dear God

Continuing conflicts, sickening strife
Deadly damning destruction
Mind-boggling misery, too much turmoil
Please excuse my cynicism
Do You have a plan for us?

Never saw or heard from You
And still believed in You
Your words, Your books, Your religions
And hoping against hope
For the elusive peace
Not to be found
Nowhere to be had

The eternal battle
Between the good and the evil
And the ensuing drama
At our expense
Do You truly tend?

Arif Ahmad

we are Your creation
So full of ourselves
Jealous, conspiring, fighting
our morals dubious, our values suspect
Your creation and imperfect

My Dear Creation
"The Response"

My Dear Creation

Now that you asked
I gave you the choice and the ability to choose
Precisely which of the two are you complaining about?

Religions are but a vehicle for peace
For unity, tolerance, and harmony
And not to assume a higher moral ground
And not a license to kill

you are My creation
Supposedly My proxy
But you assumed My role
you like being Me
you love playing God

This gift of life, this beautiful planet earth
In the grand scheme of things
Nothing more than a drop in the ocean
your narcissism, your egotism
Losing sight of the big picture
Over and over

Yes, I created you
For you are the good
your own best asset

Arif Ahmad

And you are the evil
your worst nightmare yet

And care I do
For I gave you the choice and the ability to choose
Which again of the two are you complaining about?

MANDELA

(December 2013,
on his death)

In a world torn by rift and divided by strife
What is all the fuss, all of this hoopla
From the land of the lion, we celebrate one's life
For even more relevant today is the legacy of Madiba

For prisoner number 46664 at Robben Island
His resolve to do the good, do the right
And to inspire not just his people but the entire world
In the face of ugly and unrelenting apartheid

When no one gave peace a chance to prevail
To team up with de Klerk for one Nobel Peace Prize
To turn hate into love and on such a large scale
Where do I even begin to eulogize

His lack of bitterness towards the enemy
A gentle giant, a human Everest
His humility, his humanity, his dignity, his magnanimity
And before all this, a guerrilla leader, a branded terrorist

For twenty-seven years of incarceration,
To understand and partner with the enemy in his plan
To fight hatred with forgiveness and reconciliation
In today's conflicts, we would settle for half the man

Arif Ahmad

This legend of apartheid, how can we ever forget
To breathe in the very air, exist in the same era
A soul who wielded power by letting go of it
I lived in the time of Nelson Rolihlahla Mandela

MAKING
OF A FALSE FACT

(January 2020)

pick up an idea or a statement
it does not have to be correct or verified
sure it can be against common sense or proven science
and yes, bizarre would work just fine

next, form a group of people and keep repeating it
spread it widely on social media and like-minded outlets

excessive repetition and wide dissemination are key
keep adding to the mix more of the same if need be
it works better if it stokes fear and sounds angry

and there you have it
for unsuspecting many,
a perfect false fact has been created

MAINSTREAM AMERICAN MEDIA

(December 2015)

I will start off with a joke, and please take it as just that. Though impressed with President Obama's speech on terrorism, I was amused when he challenged the Muslims and their leaders to step it up to confront extremism. It reminded me of a person on the beach who finds this bottle. He opens it, and out comes this Genie who asks the person his one wish. The person asks for a big house. The Genie rolls over laughing and says, "If I could get you a big house, would I have lived in this bottle?"

Dear President Obama, if our Muslim Genie were this good, would we have been in such a tight spot for so long?

To the real point of this writing, please allow me to start off with a few assumptions.

Mainstream Media is the face of America and rather difficult to penetrate for an outsider.

Racism, Immigration, Terrorism are real-time issues facing American society.

The group of people which comes to mind when I say Racism is Blacks.

The group of people which comes to mind when I say Immigration is Hispanics.

The group of people that come to mind when I say Terrorism is Muslims.

Now look around in the Mainstream American Media and show me the proportion of Black, Hispanic, and Muslim representation in them.

Black kids from the south side of Chicago, Hispanic and Muslim youth sitting around a table discussing these issues on CNN?

Allowing more Op-eds and Opinions.

For the better appreciation and answers may not lie without but within.

Please give us a real voice, let us in, and we might all come that much closer to the solutions.

In the true spirit of American living.

Yeah, now that's what I mean.

THE MAIN DRAW IN THIS COSMOS

(April 2015)

I watched with intent the theory of human evolution on television
The early life forms were underwater to later inhabiting land and changing into mammals
And the primates, mainly apes over time, standing up on two feet to walk and turn into humans
I agree this argument has its support in fossil records and DNA evidence
And I do not deny that there are skeletons that look half like us or that our genes are similar to that of the chimpanzees
But here is my question
Why is there not a single living proof of this transformation
Why has it stopped happening at the two ends?
Where is the family of monkeys halfway changed into humans?
Where is the family of monkeys trying to walk like us?

I believe
It started with Adam and Eve
This show and all its characters were put together for us
We are by no chance
We are the main draw in this cosmos
We are the reason for this universe
And the logical conclusion of all this
One day we would be held responsible

LOVE THIS PAIN

(March 2016)

Today we may be a nobody
Where is the silver lining in this
That kick in the guts
We have taken a few
From without and within
And this pain, this beautiful pain
The best thing to yet happen
Sure it now has our attention
Helping us gather momentum
Rising from slumber, we shall do better
Come around and be who we really are
1.6 billion weak to 1.6 billion strong
7 billion disjointed to 7 billion united
Build again from warm ashes
A greater world, a larger universe
For each and every one
We own this, love this pain
It remains much appreciated
The catalyst for our resurgence
Not a matter of if but when
And I hope it happens in time
Something I get to witness

LOTA IN CHICAGO

(May 2018)

The gift basket we all received at the recent spring APPNA (Association of Physicians of Pakistani descent of North American) meet was magnanimous and large, for, among other things, it contained a good sized, well rounded LOTA. Yes, it is not a typo. We all received a Lota (traditionally used in eastern culture for washing after defecation)

Legend has it that in one of the previous APPNA meets, there were complaints made by the Hotel administration for finding poop on the coffee pots in the rooms. Sorry everyone, this again is not a typo.

Quite often, the Men's room at ICNA and ISNA meetings is flooded.
People having visited the bathrooms on a PIA flight know what I am alluding to.

And what is the excuse for having dirty bathrooms with paper flying everywhere and water on the sink, walls, mirrors, and floor in the men's room at APPNA spring meeting evening events when there are primarily mature, Pakistani American, Muslim, Physicians in the audience?

I do not know who the perpetrators are, for sure some of us, perhaps all of us, but have we ever considered the people following us in these dirty places or the impression we make as a group on our American hosts and others.

My collective conscience at this point in time for this very issue feels ashamed.

A Piece of Me

The person doing this can hide, but we as a group just cannot.

It was our Prophet (PBUH) who said, "Cleanliness is half the faith."

I apologize, and with this, I rest my case.

LOOK PRETTY LIVING

(November 2013)

The art of Inspiring
A smile, a clap, a pat on the back
Showing the way, been there done that

The art of inspiring
A wink, a nod, a castle in the sand
An idea, a verse, a painting by hand

The art of inspiring
A child, a dream, listening to the wind
Flaws, mistakes, just about anything

The art of inspiring
In trying, in failing, and then trying again
In silence, in the soul, in our mind's domain

The art of inspiring
To risk, to chance, the courage to change
With Rumi, Iqbal and their expansive range

The art of inspiring
To fight hate with peace, with love
Our doubts and demons, let go of

The art of inspiring
To roar, laugh, cry, do your thing
I shall die trying or look pretty living

LAND OF THE PURE

(December 2013,
Pakistan on my mind)

Are you that Nation, of the Pak and Pure
With a crescent, a star, some green 'n white
Are you that Nation of character and mature
Do you have what it takes to excel 'n excite

Are you one Nation or just some people
Where at, are your motivation, your morale
Reveal your purpose, are you truly able
For you are the Nation, of Jinnah and Iqbal

Apathy no way, never your own nemesis
What goes around does come around
Stand tall and deliver on your promises
Enough of pulling each other down

I am your lost son on my ongoing journey
I am arrived, body at ease, my mind at rest
Yet I stay in your dance, in your symphony
Look around for I am still there, I never left

JAI

(September 2015)

This year's APPNA (Association of Physicians of Pakistani Descent of North America) summer meet in Orlando overlapped with August the 14th, the Independence Day of Pakistan. A fantastic get together as always it provides a good value for the time as I get to meet numerous old friends and at the same time make plenty of new ones.

There are people you connect with right away, and it was my privilege to make one such new friend in Jai, a Pakistani American Hindu Physician, an exceptionally impressive person from the outset.

It is Pakistan's Independence Day, and the atrium of this large beautiful resort is packed with throngs of people celebrating the live festivities and music. The more faithful and fun-loving crowd was up front by the stage, dancing, singing, and with Pakistani flags in hand. Green was the dominant color and feel-good the dominant mood.

A perpetual backbencher, I was soaking in fun from somewhere back there when the eyes of a friend by the stage found me, and he came back and took me forward. He gave me his Pakistani flag, and I joined this group in a state of a collective high. The energy was loud and positive, and love for our two homelands free-flowing, and at that very moment, Pakistan and America felt like, Pakista and Ameristan.

Close by, my teenage daughter, born and raised in America, and her friends were all in the same zone, and I paused for a second to appreciate that.

A Piece of Me

As I looked back at the crowd, my eyes caught Jai. There he was with his handsome face. Riding this wave of patriotism, I motioned at him to come forward. His light eyes lit up, and he obliged as I handed him my Pakistani flag that he waved around, dancing, singing, and happy to the brim.

At the end of the celebrations, he thanked me more than once, we gave each other a high five and went our ways.

Something was not right. Something was bothering my ever slowing cerebrum, but I just could not put a finger on it till finally, it dawned on me.

Why did Jai thank me so profusely?

Why did Jai, a minority Hindu Pakistani American physician among majority Muslim Pakistani American physicians on Pakistan's Independence Day being celebrated in America under the auspices of APPNA, feel the need to thank me repeatedly?

What have we done or not done to get here?

Is this my conscience, or is there more to it?

Is writing this the ownership of my share of some perceived or real guilt?

I sent Jai this writing for his permission and hope to have someday the courage and space to talk to him about this.

Someday I will cross from green into white and ask him about his life.

ISTANBUL

(July 2016, after a spate
of terrorist attacks in Istanbul)

Istanbul, Turkey, an antithesis of some of its recent unfortunate happenings, is a lovely mix of history and modernity, East and West, as it straddles two continents, Asia and Europe. Many a traveler and possibly including you have their own stories of Istanbul. This one is ours.

The year was 2003. I was doing my Physician J Visa Waiver in God's country in Northern Wisconsin. Our family of four were visiting Lahore, Pakistan, on Turkish Airline with a two-hour stopover in Istanbul.

During the flight, I remember the Turkish air hostesses coming to serve us and starting the conversation in Turkish. Awkwardly and more than once, we had to remind them that we did not speak their language. It did give us a sense of belonging, though.

We landed at Ataturk International Airport. Our connection to Lahore was leaving in two hours. Or so we thought.

As I showed up at the check-in counter, the lady looked at our still paper tickets in those days and gave us that look of, "what are you doing here, moron."

As it turned out, our connection to Lahore, which "yours truly" had booked, was not in two hours but the next day and in 26 hours. I had, one, booked us wrong, and two, not recognized my mistake till then.

It was right there, and then I realized that there was a good reason why awkward, silly, and embarrassed were conceived as words for the English language.

Once the reality sank in, I asked for our options. The flight to Lahore leaving in 2 hours was full. We were pointed towards the airport lounge, an open space with sofas, etc., where we were to spend the next 26 hours.

We tried. It was too dull, boring, and duh. To compensate for my folly, I was going to try something different.

Three of us had Pakistani passports, which made us ineligible for Turkish visas at the Airport. Only our daughter, then aged 6, was traveling on her American passport, which for $100 could get a Turkish visa stamped, but we figured it was not a good idea at her age to be out in Istanbul by herself.

We asked for the supervisor's office at the Airport and were shown to this set of rooms, which staffed several people and with one more authoritative-looking man sitting behind a desk. Having introduced ourselves, I tried selling him our story and my mistake. I then made our plea.

Is there any way we can get out and spend a day in Istanbul?

There was some language barrier, but the officer, a no-fuss, kind-looking person, asked me to get a Turkish visa stamped on our daughter's American passport. This I happily did, still not sure where it was all headed.

He then asked for all our Pakistani Passports and put them on a shelf in his office. He then showed us this door on the side and said, outside this door is Istanbul, see you tomorrow.

It was there, and then I realized that there was a good reason elated, liberated, and wow were added to the English language as words.

And just like that, we stepped out to this beauty of a city called Istanbul. The next 24 hours, we traveled, ate, shopped, and celebrated this fun-filled, unexpected visit to this world-class destination. No passports, no visas, no problem.

We soaked in the majesty of the blue mosque. We walked the brick-laden old city. We taxied around this city of rolling hills with mosques on top, which are shown lights at night and look amazingly beautiful and we constantly amused ourselves with a lot of dizzying zeroes behind everything as the exchange rate of Lira to USD in those days was in millions.

And yes, we were again spoken to in Turkish a few more times, which made us feel at home and, well, somewhat Turkish, I guess.

As many of you can relate to, Istanbul, Turkey, remains a city, a country, a people par excellence. God willing, I would love to go back someday for my second visit. Meanwhile, to the city which made us feel at home, I say, stay strong and in peace, Amen.

IN OUR CITIES OF TODAY

(March 2017)

With a purpose and eager steps
I head back into the woods
For that experience
I seem never to get enough of
How the place goes hush,
with eyes on me, I feel and don't see,
till I settle down,
for my turn,
and wait for it to come alive,
Slowly
Birds, red and blue,
now all around me
Passing geese honk hi
Glancing doves whistle by

An eagle with intent, circling the pasture
The loud and rowdy woodpecker,
just yards away at eye level
And two feet from my two feet,
munching on clover is a rabbit

Gliding squirrels,
grey, blonde and tan,
own the floor, the trees, and the space in between
And yes, the deer,
ever nervous, all attentive, turning ears

Arif Ahmad

As the doe courageously steps out in the open,
the dark shadow of a buck stands still and watching from well inside the tree line

Leaves changing colors,
dancing to the tune of their own rainbow
A distant coyote's Aaaoouuuuu
An owl's ouu, ouu, u, oouuuuuu

A feeding flock of turkeys,
ladies, longbeards, young ones,
a few yelps and clucks, an occasional gobble
Ignoring me, allowing me, in spite of me
The camaraderie, the harmony

As I grow into this ecosystem
They accept me as one of them
Tolerate me for who I am
And I can stay
For as long as,
I keep to myself, sit still and out of their way
Something I struggle to find in our cities of today

I LOVE THE FOURTEENTH OF AUGUST

(August 14, 1947 is the Independence
Day of Pakistan)

My one hand is repeatedly stabbing me in the chest
The fingers of the other are trying to plug those gaping, gushing gashes
My one leg is busy kicking me in the guts
The other one is dragging, refusing to walk with
Yet there is optimism, there is hope
For my heart is still in it
My mind is still working
But for that small matter
Of them hating each other
Deja vu
Awkward, good for nothing
Dysfunctional all right
I am hurting, struggling, barely moving
Who am I kidding
Is this some weird dream
Is this really happening
I love the fourteenth of August
I hate August the fourteenth

HELLO SILVER

(July 2014)

What!
Old, me, ever
Way later, perhaps never
Or so I thought
But here it is, in a flash
In just about all its splendor,
experience in for prowess, glory without fanfare
With all the aches and pains
The creaking and cracking
Slowly finding place, setting in
Chipping away and eroding
Lines receding
Lines bulging

As the disconnect between the mind and the body grows,
"Say hello to silver, Say hi to wrinkles"
Love it or hate it, ready or not,
Get a grip AA
The once unthinkable is happening and here to stay

AGING
Undeniable, Unrelenting
You Beauty

AMERICANS ARE PITTED AGAINST ONE ANOTHER

(February 2018,
published by the AP)

Irrespective of the merits of the released Nunes memo or its rebuttal in the yet unreleased Schiff memo, the end results are the same.

These have to be good times for the enemies of America for collusion or no collusion, obstruction of justice or not, does it really matter?
The end results are the same.

Americans pitched against Americans, the State fighting with its own institutions, a severe test of the American democracy and way of life, precisely as our foes would have planned and wished upon us.

Irrespective of whatever transpires next, the goals of American adversaries are being achieved in real and present time. This has hurt, is hurting, and is likely to keep hurting for a while yet.

HAJJ, GO FOR IT

(September 2017 – Dedicated to all who inspired
and guided us and hoping this will do the same for others)

Behind me in line getting on the bus to the airport was this big heavy set guy, reeking of alcohol, unsteady on his feet. His belly touched me. I moved away with an, excuse me. He again drifted closer. A little irritated, I said, excuse me again, pulled Farah and myself out of the line and let him get ahead. Is this my introduction to patience? Oh boy. This may be a long two weeks.

Tentative, unsure, nervous is how I would describe my feelings. A day before leaving, I felt a little heavy and dragging some. Farah and I were heading out for Hajj. It is sweltering there, 100 F plus, millions of people, the smell, the sounds, dirty bathrooms, surely it would be a nightmare and especially with my baggage. I repeatedly prayed for ease and grace. I was not sure of either.

Hajj is a once in a lifetime mandatory ritual for all physically and financially able Muslims. I was reasonably trained and had a plan in place. S is for smile, P is for patience. You are at Hajj. I was tested right at the beginning getting on the bus, and I got some irritated. I failed early on and doubled down on my resolve to do better.

Chicago, New York, Medina went smoothly. We got out in a reasonable time from the airport. Medina is where Prophet Muhammad, peace be upon him, is buried along with many of his companions and family. Got there at Asr time and rushed to Masjid Nabawi (Prophet Muhammad's Mosque and burial place, Roza) for prayers.

A Piece of Me

I had previously visited Riadhul Jannah (the green-carpeted part of Masjid Nabwi, called a part of paradise with heightened significance for prayers) in Umrah and was sure and ready that it was not going to happen this time around with the high Hajj traffic. Except for the kid in me. After Asr prayers, I tried getting in line for the Roza without success. The guard waved me towards the line for Riadhul Jannah, a little smaller which as you exit leads to the Roza.

In the line, I got talking to a black young man about 6 inches taller than and in front of me. I asked him a question to try and refresh my memory of the place. As we were talking and moving forward, he made room effortlessly with his presence, and I would just fill up the space he was creating behind him. Another person behind me, his first time there, started asking me about the place and where which made me feel some important and relevant. A couple of minutes later, I looked down, and I was standing on the green carpet, just like that. In Riadhul Jannah, I try to keep it short, so others can use the limited space and walked out by the Roza, paying my respects, all this within the first hour of being in Medina.

Such hospitality and without much difficulty or effort. I just could not stop crying. That is the beauty of this trip. The tears usually have a mind of their own. Welcome to Medina.

In Masjid Nabawi, I am like a kid in a candy store. This is a beautiful mosque in more than one way, and I just cannot have my fill. At times I would just stand watching, admiring. Other times I would imagine going back in time and watch history unfold. On another occasion, I ventured to the roof. Compared to the air-conditioned and comfortably carpeted ground floor, the roof is tiled and must have been 90F even at night. It was beautiful and empty except for this one guy who sat there, prayer rug laid out, Quran in hand, and with a view of the Green Dome and the Minaret. I walked up to him and told him he had the best seat in the house. I am not sure if he understood.

Most of the Hajj groups had already left. The last day before we left Medina, it felt we had the Masjid to ourselves. I had my fill if there is ever such a thing.

Prophet Muhammad, peace be upon him, was unable to read or write. Yes, he was illiterate. He was given the Quran, a book which does not cease to amaze for the wisdom it holds. Medina is a welcoming place, always kind, always sweet. My unease had eased off some, though not completely. Surely Mecca with the rituals (Manasik) is where we would get hit hard with all kinds of difficulty.

Day one of the rituals was an early start from Medina to Jeddah and then to Mecca wearing two white unstitched sheets, the Ihram. Over the next few days, the Manasik with Umrah (Tawaf, Saee), Arafat, Muzdalifah, Mina, Stoning, Tawaf, cutting of hair, Mina, Stoning, Tawaf, etc.

Arafat is the main part of Hajj. It was kind to us with gathering clouds, winds, and rain that afternoon, which made our stay and commute to Muzdalifah all that easy. The move to Muzdalifah only took 2 hours where we fell asleep after the prayers. Mina was comfortable. Stoning with the large crowds well managed. The Tawafs were a labor of love with that magical house Kaaba in full view. Saee was soothing, knowing that all the Muslims were following in the footsteps of an Egyptian slave girl. Getting out of the Ihram, shaving of the head, and a shower was an enjoyable treat, something to look forward to. We were able to check all the boxes. It was a spiritual, physical, and mental boot camp more so anticipatory than in reality.

One night in Mina, I went for a walk outside our camp. There were people everywhere, on the footpaths, entire families, and seemingly very happy and content. I returned a more humble and appreciative person.

We had no hardships at all. Nothing untoward, nothing we could not handle. The logistics and surroundings were good. The much-anticipated difficulties never occurred. The crowds were a miracle of their own. These massive unrehearsed hoards of people from all over the World kept doing the rituals in a very organized manner. The expected issues and fears never materialized.

Between the rituals and prayers, one is always short on sleep, but halfway through, I felt a wind beneath my wings, which carried me through. It felt as if on cruise control. Things were happening without putting in too much effort. By this time, my fears were replaced by an unexplainable sense of tranquility and peace. Farah, in parallel, was doing even better than me. Always a step or two ahead of me, I was struggling to keep up with her. Once I tried to take it easy at the prayer time and not go to the Masjid, and she would have no part of it, and I am so glad for that.

The scenes stay with you. A bent-over old, hand in hand, couple crossed us at double our speed during Tawaf. You lift your hands for prayers, and you see Kaaba across them. Like a movie trailer, I could see the clip of the day of judgment with the masses, except that I could separate myself some with my status in this World, but that day shall be a different story.

On our way back, I was a doctor to several sick companions. The husband of one of them asked me. What is your secret? Why are you not ill and still so upbeat? He caught me off guard. I did not have a good answer and just shrugged my shoulders.

Then as I thought it over, it dawned on me. The experience of Hajj is irrespective of the social status or the country you come from. There were people doing all the Hajj on foot and seemed very excited and content. There were individuals with no shade or comfort by the roadside and seemingly happy just to be there, to be able to do Hajj. It is all about your attitude. I repeat, it is all about your attitude, and the plan made out for you is based on that. The first big guy at the very beginning who irritated me brushed up my preparation with S for Smile and P for Patience. The second one at Masjid Nabawi walked me into Riadhul Jannah, easing my stress and tension.

I also learned that for those few weeks, the journey is the destination. When the going is easy, you remember God, for you are at Hajj. When it is not very easy, you remember God, for you are at Hajj. Praying looking at Kaaba, eating, sleeping, waiting in line, all the time you are at Hajj, in attendance with God and the Giants of history. Many of the Manasik, most of us, would only do once in our lifetime, so enjoy for you are at Hajj.

Now that I look back, I believe that at Hajj, you are a guest and your host is God and the Prophet. Your experience and how you are received depends on the kind of guest you are, the effort you are putting in, and the will to back it up. The more you try to be a good guest, the better you will be received, and the greater your experience shall be. This is the biggest miracle of Hajj. I guarantee you this.

GOLDEN EMBOLDEN

(May 2017. Little did I know where
it would end up on January 6, 2021)

APPNA is the Association of Physicians of Pakistani Descent of North America, of which I am a member.
Today I woke up to this e-Newsletter from APPNA and its President.
It sadly mentions two ongoing issues.

1- Increased vetting of APPNA physicians returning home after traveling abroad and including a past APPNA President to a point where many are now reluctant to travel outside of the USA.
2- Decrease in training and residency visas for overseas physicians, many of whom have invested years and a substantial amount of money going through the process and exams, and when there is a clear and present shortage of the same in America.

My mood went south on reading all this. I thought about my options.
1- Curl up and go to sleep.
2- It is not affecting me, stay out of it.
3- Go on with my day and try and lift up my spirits.

But closing my eyes would not make the dilemma go away.
Too much of this is happening and too close to home.
Houston, we have a problem.

We at APPNA are no schmucks.
This is not Timbuktu but the United States of America in the year 2017.
This is happening to American physicians and wannabes.

Arif Ahmad

Am I some worried today for writing all this?
Yes, for sure.
And no, I refuse to be intimidated and or live in fear.
This is my country, and I am going to own it with all its blessings and ills.

This brings me to the phenomenon of Golden embolden.
The direct or indirect influence of President Trump on fellow Americans.
With all its good and bad.
Imposed or implied,
and unfortunately with some hatred and discord.

Has President Golden emboldened some Americans to mistreat and demean fellow Americans in subtle and not so subtle ways?
Are personal and civil rights being encroached upon?
Is there growing color intolerance?
I sure hope not, but there are far too many cries of injustice and travesties to call it a coincidence.

President Trump, you are the one most responsible for your legacy and all of this.
As your predecessor rightly said, the buck stops with you.
The hole some emboldened are digging for other Americans would be for all of us to climb out of.
These cries are still easy to ignore, though they are getting louder.
I wish you the very best, for we are in this together.

May the gracious and better shades of Gold shine on all of us for generations to come.

Amen.

GOLDEN AGE

(June 2014)

I had rather burn the school down than tolerate this. I heard it loud and clear.

I was standing outside my high school Principal's office in a long dim corridor, which felt colder than usual with its always cement floors, high ceilings, and painted walls. The hanging black and white framed pictures of various classes with their teachers were all staring at me. I wanted to run away and keep running.

Welcome to St. Anthony High School, Lahore, Pakistan. I was 15; the year was 1978.

I was born to middle-class parents in Lahore, Pakistan. We had some and had to wait and plan for some more. The one thing I was blessed with not getting shortchanged was my education. My first three years of schooling was coeducation at Sacred Heart, a Catholic missionary school run by Irish white-robed Sisters and Mothers. In those days, the girls would stay and finish grade 10 at the same school, whereas the boys would separate at year four and transfer to nearby St. Anthony High School, another Catholic missionary school with a Church on-premises but run by Irish white-robed Brothers and Fathers instead.

Both these schools are located at a walking distance on the opposite side of the majestic Mall Road, the main boulevard of Lahore, with a nostalgic mix of oversized colonial age buildings exuding old-world charm and modern architecture displaying eastern grace intermingled with hundreds of acres of lush green parks and old massive shadowy trees laden recreational spaces.

If names were a flavor, then you can try and savor some of the institutions situated along the Mall such as Lahore Zoo, Lahore Museum, Punjab University, Lahore High Court, Governor house, Bagh-e-Jinnah, Wapda (Federal electricity department where my father worked), State Bank of Pakistan, Alhamra Art Center and Lahore Gymkhana. I spent a considerable portion of my early years in this rustic domain and, thanks to Google search and maps, still virtually transport myself to this area often.

Brother Golden, in his flowing white robes, was our Principal at St. Anthony. I am not sure if he was more white than red or otherwise, but I am very sure that his personality was unambiguous, a very tough discipline-oriented person who would cane us for being late to school, yell and point at us for indiscipline and yes froth at the corners of his mouth when angry. He was a brisk walker between points A and B and hence the flowing white robes. Though a palpable apprehension of fear was never far off, the school ran like a well-oiled machine offering top-notch education at a still subsidized and affordable fee for the masses.

I had crossed paths with Brother Golden before. Once I was late for school. It was a winter morning, and I was in shorts, so I must have been in the lower grades, I believe 5th. There were a few of us lined up in the front school ground. He approached each one of us, and we were expected to present him with our right hand. I did just that, and the cane zinged and brushed the tips of my fingers. He moved on as I started blowing into and rubbing my numb fingers.

Another time, batting in a cricket match on a matting wicket in the school ground at the back, I pulled a ball which bounced and broke through a classroom door glass panel. I was called up and scolded.

We were in Grade 10, Mr. Rizvi's class. This was the last year of High School, matriculation, followed hopefully by two years of college and then medical school, that is, if everything fell into place and there were no mishaps. I was a good student, never in the top one or two in class but always in the top ten percent. I also had a rebel in me, from sports of all kinds I could put my hands on to mischief and fun, often being the planner and executioner in chief. If daring and attending uninvited wedding ceremonies for free good food sounds interesting, then that was me.

Now to be fair to me, those were the days with black and white television with one channel only and before cell phones, the internet, and computers. I lived my life outside and in the fast lane though there were limits. I was not into girls, alcohol, drugs, and not even smoking, which, although I may have tried a couple of cigarettes growing up, never developed a liking for or took up to look cool. I was plenty cool without all this, or so I thought. Ha.

Our class ten was on the second floor, the front end of the two-story red brick school building. We were probably around forty some students in each class. Something was happening to me around that time. It was a mindset thing. Out of nowhere, I started feeling like an adult, as if I was on top of the world and with not many things able to hold me back. In my sight was the around the corner liberty with college life with a motorbike and to be able to come and go at will. It felt like I owned the world and was about to declare that.

The planner-in-chief in me came up with an idea. What if the entire class bunked school for one day and went to the movies. I ran my idea by my besties, and lo and behold, we were on to it. The plan was to be dropped at school just as always but then not come to class but instead walk out to a nearby cinema. We started spreading the word around in between classes. In one particular class, I stood at the door to share this plan with all the boys one by one and before the teacher showed up. After another class, I walked up to the front to announce and invite. Now, remember I was 15 and still commuted on bus and foot. St. Anthony, meanwhile, was a full-time blue blazer, striped tie, blue shirt, and grey trousers school, without permission to be anywhere outside or else during the school hours. St. Anthony High School, Lahore was Brother Golden's turf.

Planned, performed, and waiting on execution, fingers crossed, the next day, about half the class showed up at the theater. We came to the school, as usual, dropped by our parents or the bus. Instead of coming to the morning assembly line up we stayed and gathered outside the school premises. The macho gang then walked to the theater as we were still below the legal driving age. I felt initially puzzled and then embarrassed to find out that the cinema only ran evening shows. We still had a point to prove, and so we putzed around, ate, and finally went back to school after the final bell and mixed up with the crowd of students coming out and to go home just like another day. Except it was not just another day, and the following days were not going to be either.

We showed up at school the next day as if nothing had happened. We pretended to be calm and normal except that our surroundings were not. The rumor was that the word was out, and a puny little classmate of ours, Khawar, had given out our plan under threat and duress. We were asked to report to the Principal's office and with our parents.

And there I was, standing in that corridor outside Brother Golden's office with my father inside with him when I heard him growl. I had rather burn the school down than tolerate this. I heard father say something in a lower pitch, then some discussion back and forth, which I could not make up.

As I stood and waited outside, a cold shudder ran through my body, and my mind felt detached as if in a zone of its own. My entire life till then and its promise to become a physician, a big deal in those pre-computer days, flashed in front of me. What if I was expelled and my efforts till then and my potential cut short? What about my role model, good boy reputation? My future at that very point was out of my hands, and "burn the school down" line had made me acutely aware of that.

The wait lasted about 15 minutes, which felt like hours, and after which I was called inside. I pulled open the double panel white painted doors and walked in.

A Piece of Me

Though I had peeked inside this part open door walking in the administration hallway at times, this was the first time I had been inside Brother Golden's office. The room was dimly lit, spacious, and almost a square with the same high ceilings. The two large windows were covered with curtains, with one pulled just enough to let in a streak of sunlight, which gave me a strange feeling of hope.

Brother Golden sat on his chair with his back towards the windows. Father sat at one of the two chairs across the large wooden desk. A green desk lamp was the other source of light in the room. I walked in and stood as far as I could get away from the side of the desk to the left of Brother Golden and right of my father and waited obediently.

Father started the conversation. He spoke to me about my mistake and that it cannot be repeated. I stood there silent, my mind phasing in and out, waiting in apprehension to be told that I was done. Brother Golden, for the most part, stayed quiet, poker-faced, staring down straight at the desk. I believe this was new for him too, he looked a little uncomfortable, out of place. At one point, he looked up to me and said, "small moments can change a life forever, your potential is better than this."

I was feeling better already. The feeling of impending doom was receding. He leaned over and handed father a paper, a written apology. Father read the paper, signed it, and waved at me to sit in the second chair across the desk to the right of him. He gave me the paper to read and sign. I looked at the paper, pretended to read, maybe even tried, my eyes and mind not wanting to read or comprehend, and signed the paper anyway to get it over with. To this day, I have no idea what exactly was written that I signed. Today it feels as if the phrase, a slap on the wrist, was invented that day.

I never asked, and father never told me the conversation he had with Brother Golden.

Suffice it to say that I graduated with flying colors, went to college with my mischievous bone still intact though toned down some, and ended up being a physician and a cardiologist in the USA. There was warning enough but no lingering repercussions or scars for me or any of the culprits. We were not maltreated by any of the staff and teachers for the rest of our time at St. Anthony. As a matter of fact, no one, including my father, ever reminded me of this again.

I would still run into Brother Golden on the school premises, the man of few words he was, seemed gentler with me. I would even break into a short exchange of pleasantries with him, something very unusual by his standards. Good morning Sir. Hello, he would nod back with a hint of a smile. How is the cricket team doing, he would ask? Sir, we are progressing well in the inter-school tournament. He probably knew that already. Good day Sir. He would nod and smile back and keep walking. In those last few months and for the first time in years, I saw him smile.

Brother Golden left St. Anthony High a few months before I graduated. He was my Principal for almost all of the seven years I was there. He was replaced by Father Donnelly who I am quoting from a letter he gave me at graduation dated May 25th, 1979.
"Thanks to an interest in study and considerable aptitude for it, he has consistently gained excellent results.
One of the school's most outstanding sportsmen.
He has impressed his teachers with his maturity, courtesy and bearing and his high standard of conduct and behavior."

High standard of conduct and behavior?

I remain a St. Anthonian forever. Brother Golden remains a part of the person I am. Anyone who visits me in my office today notices one thing right away. It is dimly lit, with the curtains pulled apart just enough to let in a streak of sunlight.

GOD AND INCLUSIVENESS

(August 2017)

The star-studded skies, a prairie full of life, remind me of God and inclusiveness each time. As we embark on Hajj in submission to God, here are some lines from across several faiths in this light.

Talbiyah (the prayer of Hajj, a once in a lifetime mandatory pilgrimage to Mecca for financially and physically able Muslims)

Labbayka Allahumma labbayk, labbayka laa shareeka laka labbayk. Inna al-hamd wa'l-ni'mata laka wa'l-mulk, laa shareeka lak
(Here I am, O Allah, here I am. Here I am, You have no partner, here I am. Verily all praise and blessings are Yours, and all sovereignty, You have no partner.)

1 Thessalonians 2:12 (New Testament)
Encouraging, comforting, and urging you to live lives worthy of God, who calls you into his kingdom and glory.

Hebrews 11:1 (New Testament)
Now faith is confidence in what we hope for and assurance about what we do not see

Jeremiah 32:27 (Old Testament)
"I am the LORD, the God of all mankind. Is anything too hard for me?"

Surah Al-Fatihah, Quran (Islam)
Praise be to Allah, the Lord of all the Worlds.

Shvetashwataro Upanishad (ancient Sanskrit text, Hinduism)
(There is) just one divinity, manifestly hidden everywhere
Pervading everything, the soul of every living creature.
The one that directs the actions of all and lives across all times.
Witness to everything, pure and perfect, devoid of all (worldly) qualities and attributes. -

Buddha (Buddhism)
"Be kind to all creatures; this is the true religion."

Guru Nanak (Sikhism)
"Those who have loved are those that have found God."

FUNDAMENTALLY ONE

(April 2017)

For all of our blood spilling differences,
How so different are we really?
The anatomy taught in medical schools,
Is it different for Muslims, Christians, and Jews?
Don't we all have the same workings, the same physiology?
The same disease processes, the same pathology?
Or does the appendix lay different for a Shia from a Sunni?
Or the neurons in the brain transmit differently?
Does cancer affect an Indian and spare a Pakistani?
Or Russians have two and Americans just one kidney?
Does aspirin work differently for a Palestinian and an Israeli?
That blood on the ground still some wet,
Is their's red and them's mahogany?
For sure, the heart is where the difference has to be.
Well, not really,
For I doctor the heart, and that is something I have yet to see.
So if all shades of skin are the same within,
Why such hate and to this extreme?
To me, it does seem akin,
To darn our own self and damn our own being.
For we can hurt, we can kill, to our want, to our will,
And keep playing havoc,
On this tiny planet, this pale blue dot.
When all is said and done,
We remain "Fundamentally One"

FROM BEHIND THE MASK

(August 2020)

From behind the mask, I try, smiling, nodding, looking for a response, and uncertain if mine was received or the other person returned, for such is the life with the mask and this very American tradition.

The other day a colleague helped some by saying, I know you're smiling behind that mask.

So much of the American way depends on acknowledging and greeting passersby, the ones we know, and perfect strangers.

The masked living has taken a bite out of this tradition, at a time of stress compounded by added factors, when this gesture of goodwill is needed the most. A simple reflex ritual has become a bit of an effort.

As crucial as it is to wear till the vaccine arrives, may short live the mask and long live this American tradition.

FRESH TRACKS

(December 2020)

Why I would extend my left arm for the Covid-19 vaccine and why it is a great American story but with a caveat.

As a physician, I practice medicine, a science of probabilities. There is no outcome absolute or 100% guaranteed or implied. We do, however, strive through trials and research to increase the odds of the desired result. Our goal is that the pros outweigh the cons. Such appears to be the case with the Covid-19 vaccine. Please consider that taking Tylenol may have potential side effects also.

So far, the Covid-19 vaccine has made a great American story. Already two 95% effective vaccines developed and with rapid speed when failure was not an option. The vaccine's delivery is based on merit with the health care staff and the high-risk population upfront.

The caveat is the question of the availability of this vaccine to the developing nations and with what speed and priority?

Thus when it is my turn, I would gladly roll up my sleeve and extend my proud brown American left arm for the Covid-19 vaccine, as I am right-handed. I am also acutely aware of this American privilege not based on race, color, class, or wealth and hoping we meet these goals within and globally.

This is our chance to smile and shine for the history books, yet again.

FOR THE SAKE OF HEAVENS, FOR HEAVEN'S SAKE

(July 2014 – The Israeli-Palestinian Conflict)

The World bleeds around this most chronic ill
The mother of all conflicts
For such little space, a tiny area on the map
The history of hatred is mind-boggling
The central issue, the bottom line, is NOT ENOUGH LAND,
LAND, which the World can help create over the sea
Or little some the expansive neighbors can graciously add

If Abraham was to come alive today
Would he not gather his entire family and probably say
"Do it over, do it better, step it up."
"Come on people, get your act together, enough is enough."
Albeit
Would his say in this day still carry any weight?

Moses, Jesus, Muhammad
How do I feel they are faring up there?
How do you think they are holding out?
Content, ecstatic, full of joy?
Or disappointed, dejected, thoroughly annoyed?

You are so wrong, I am so right
And together, we create
For the sake of heavens, for heaven's sake

A Piece of Me

Unending bloodshed, this never-ending plight
Never pausing, never thinking
That at the end of the day
It is the same genes, the same blood on both sides of the aisle
One Big Unhappy Family
Where misery is shared, and so is destiny

FOR ALL ITS CRITICISM

(November 2018)

the culmination of the moment of fair chase hunting
our American pride, the whitetail deer king
of friends, the earth, the experience, the fellowship
without wings or legs
climbing, staying stealth
25 feet up in the tree
archery at close quarters is never easy
the meat going to the local food pantry
yes, you read that right
the meat serving local Americans food inadequate, protein deficient, and hungry
and some deer kabobs for you and me

ENOUGH

(March 2017, Pakistan
suffering from terrorism)

Done and dusted
Left for dead
We are back up on our feet
Kicking, fighting
Showing our resolve, our grit
That stuff we are made of
And the oomph we got left

Besides our lingering fears
Beyond our worst nightmares
A psyche mutilated, a generation terrorized
Our back up against the wall
Wounded, cornered
Repeatedly wronged
Scarred beyond recognition
At the edge of oblivion
The push has come to shove
Enough
And we march on as one
A nation united
Love us or hate our guts
but make no mistake about it
This is when we'll give it our all
Now is when we do our best

DISTRACTED

(October 2019, inside APPNA)

once upon a time
several hundred
fond of politics
campaigns, canvassing
elections
I was one of them
just as wrong
just as dumb

we kept bleeding
expanding the fault lines
at the center
alumni and chapters
scarred history everywhere
cruelty of the highest order
we kept serving each other
over and over

inbreeding riddance
delivered us
this Frankenstein monster
more positions
more conflicts
more to fight for
amongst mere hundreds

best of mates
now sworn enemies

A Piece of Me

feeding the same crap
expecting different results
half of us already,
some kinda boss
the other half in a race,
for yet another office

our perpetual leaders
hopping between positions,
to the tune of drag down music,
with an unending supply of chairs
Arif, don't bash our leaders
what we feed them
is what they become

these elections
deceit and lies
candidates, voters
supporters
losing friends
out of sync,
with what we can
out of touch,
with what we must
losing our worth
for what

can we
simplify this mess
get out of these
self-depreciating madness
shrink our governance
only a few hundred
less is
more for us

DEAR MR. DONALD TRUMP

(November 2015, little did I know)

Are you really happening?

I thought long and hard about taking you up. I asked myself if I should even take someone who carries whatever that thing is on your shoulders seriously. The answer was obvious. I had to do this for all our children.

First, it was the Hispanics and now the Muslims. I find your comments on the American Muslim database and closing of the Mosques in poor taste, though probably a good reflection of your person and personality.

Not only was the question and your answer Un-American but let me make something very clear to you right at the outset. As much as you exude inequality, please, for a minute, do not think that you are any more American than any other law-abiding citizen.

If anything, such questions and comments only polarize the society more and create layers of citizenships the exact breeding grounds for the misery which at the breaking point of some souls is called extremism, the worst form of which is terrorism.

Actually, tell me a little more about your forefathers. Were they looking for a better life, fleeing persecution, why really did they come to America? How were they welcomed? Has any of the Trumps ever committed a crime, and if yes, does that make all Trumps criminal?

I believe you are a decoy. A person who is creating so much damage in his path that it will make your opponent run away with the race. The disservice you are doing to your party and its ideals is probably beyond repair in the short term, at least.

Not only this, you are hurting the very basic fabric of this country. You are so not American and pro-anarchy, chaos and terrorism. You are a terrorist's best-case scenario, for you shall increase the breeding grounds several fold.

You divert energies away from the real issues by assuming that all lives are not equal. You are a symbol of what America is not, a cocky, rude, obnoxious, disrespectful, and distasteful billionaire. Please remind me to remove this last line from my final draft as I am trying my best not to stoop down to your level of decency.

Shame on you and your thought processes.

Enough. Please.

Let me also educate you about Islam in one line. Like any other faith, Islam is just as good as the majority of its followers and just as poor as its deviants and distractors, and yes, it has nothing to do with the price of tea in China.

And yes, as long as you keep unloading such misery and then some more, deviant response, extremism and terrorism are going to keep flourishing, and that is probably why so far all the King's men and all the King's horses have been unable to put Humpty Dumpty together again.

So to our equal American children, I say, be as much pro-Islam, pro-all religions or no religion, pro-America, pro-world, pro-humanity, pro-universe as you want and wish.
You all go and drown this world in good.

Best always.
Arif Ahmad

CHILDREN WILL BE CHILDREN

(December 2014, Pershawar, Thar, Newtown)

How do we tell children apart?
Our children from those less privileged?
Our children from those of a terrorist?
Hungry children from sick children?
Pretending to play dead children, from dead children?

How in the hell do they tell?
Which one to let live, which one to kill?

Reactive governance, absent strategy?
Politics of war, political warring?
Failing diplomacy, content apathy?
In a burden we all share
This child play is for real
There, here, elsewhere, anywhere
Children will be children, they are dying everywhere

Paying the price, laying their lives
Crying out loud then going quiet
Our past, our present, haunting our future
Children are children, they are dying everywhere

Is there something wrong with this picture?
How is this not our mutual shame?
How is this not our shared failure?
Children, our children, are dying everywhere

BUT WAIT A SECOND

(January 2017)

Radical Islamic terrorists, we don't want them here, says the POTUS.
Agreed, Mr. President, and thank you so very much for protecting us.
But wait a second.
Name me one country which does.
And I hate to break it to you that radical Islamic terrorism is our baby.
Do wars in Afghanistan, Al-Qaeda, and Iraq, ISIS, ring a bell.
And now we close our doors for all their victims to stay in hell.
Well, well, well.

BOSA OF HAJR-E-ASWAD
(KISSING OF THE BLACK STONE)

(January 2014)

For the umpteenth time, I was close to the Hajr-e-Aswad, the Black Stone only a few feet away, as I stood watching, thinking, and hoping against hope. The struggling mass of humans with the chaotic pushing and shoving was in full swing, a show of raw force like none I had experienced before.

Finally decided, disappointed and discouraged, I moved away from the emotionally charged crowd, which was fiercely and physically engrossed in the ritual of attempting to kiss the Black Stone. The reality that the evasive Bosa or the Kiss was not going to happen for me was sinking in, and so be it.

This was my first visit to The Kaaba, the House of God, built by Abraham in Mecca, a simple yet one of the most beautiful and elegant structures I have ever laid my eyes on. I sat admiring, I stood awestruck, and I walked mesmerized by the majestic grace of a structure so uncomplicated.

Hajr-e-Aswad, the black stone from paradise, is on one of its corners. Touching and kissing the stone, following in the footsteps of Prophet Muhammad (peace be upon him), though not mandatory, is highly preferable and one of the most physically challenging rituals of Hajj and Umrah. Throw in an intensely passionate crowd of several hundred in the space of several feet and from all directions and every one of them wanting to kiss the stone, and one can begin to understand the struggle.

A Piece of Me

I had completed my other rituals with relative ease but was on the verge of giving up on the elusive Bosa of Hajr-e-Aswad. My saving grace was that it was not for the lack of will or want, but for my refusal to wrestle my way in to do that.

Most of the other rituals are performed with some discipline, a credit to hundreds of thousands of people from different nationalities, speaking different languages, and no prior rehearsals. However, the Bosa of Hajr-e-Aswad stirs emotions like nothing else, and the wheels do come off the wagon of discipline here.

The word going around is that people have lost their lives with suffocation or getting trampled to fulfill this ritual. Even though pushing and thrusting are forbidden to the extent that the entire ritual may lose its value in front of God, the practice continues.

Once or twice my hormones toyed with the idea of taking on the challenge and getting involved with the conglomerate of bodies and forcing my way in, thankfully to be overridden by good common sense out of the upper chamber.

Being in the House of God, asking the Almighty to let me have the Kiss was an option. The risk was the disappointment of a prayer gone begging as the task was daunting at the least and impossible at the worse.

What transpired next is my story, my own little miracle, and there are plenty of them going around at that place.

As it happened, I was sitting on one side of the Kaaba when with some inkling, I got up and got in the swing of Tawaf, which is the counterclockwise walking around the Kaaba in circles. I remember looking at the Kaaba and wishing for the coveted Kiss. It was a silent, half prayer at best, a defense mechanism in that, if not fulfilled, would not disappoint me.

I next noticed three young men right in front of me in Ihram, the two white sheets worn by men. I remember the one on the left with a handsome and kind face and probably in his thirties. The men looked at each other with a meaningful gaze and nodded. Next, they started walking towards the Black Stone, Hajr-e-Aswad. Right behind them and instinctively, I followed.

As they arrived in the general area of the Black Stone, they stood still, hands by their sides, held their ground, and started chanting the words, "No Pushing, Please No Pushing, No Pushing." Two other people already there and to my right joined in with "Dhakka Nahin, Dhakka Nahin," which in Urdu means the same, "No Pushing." By now, I had joined the group and was feverishly repeating, no pushing, no pushing, no pushing, please.

Few more people joined us from behind and with the same slogan. At this point, we were probably about ten people chanting "No Pushing" and just holding our place passively in the crowd, which by now had dramatically calmed down.

The group was so tight that as the person in front, having kissed the stone, moved out, the rest of the group got pulled in, and I kept getting closer. Next, I was at an arm's length from the Black Stone.

Knowing very well that one large push from the crowd could throw me out of my place, I touched the stone first with one hand and then the other. If the Kiss did not materialize, at least I had the stone felt.

The very next moment, I was right in front of the stone and with the back of a woman's head, the only thing in between. My biggest worry at this point was to miss the Kiss after literally being inches from the Hajr-e-Aswad. The woman, it seemed, was in no rush.

My first instinct was to grab her head and move it out of my way. Grab the woman's head, I did. I then fought the ugly urge of pushing her head away and instead waited nervously. Finally, as she moved out of the way, I bent and kissed the stone once only, and in literally a second, it was all over. I then moved out swiftly to make way for others.

Just before the Kiss, as I got close to the Hajr-e-Aswad, I must have been in a zone of some sort as my mind had blocked out the surrounding sights and sounds. I say this because I cannot recall the later chanting or hearing of the "No Pushing" slogan, and neither do I remember seeing any of those men again.

That I shared the story of this miracle of some sort in my life is a small personal matter. A better wish is if the Muslims from all over the world can somehow come together and perform this ritual in an orderly manner and with discipline and civility.

That the Bosa of Hajr-e-Aswad becomes available to the elderly, the weak, the women alike would be the next frontier, a challenge worth writing, dreaming, and praying for.

For my lack of conviction, it might just be a silent, half a prayer, though, just so I do not feel denied if this one miracle never happens.

AN ATYPICAL PITCH TO EXERCISE

(November 2013)

My goal with this writing is to inspire you to exercise. I am going to try to do this in a rather atypical manner.

With that being said, if you exercise and do it regularly, then this writing is not for you. You can stop here and do something else with your time. If you do not exercise or not regularly enough, please keep reading and for your own sake.

You probably know everything there is to know about exercise. The only scientific data I will share is that most of us are likely to suffer and die from either heart-related issues or some form of cancer, and lack of regular physical exercise is now shown to be one of the biggest risk factors for them.

I would like you to understand two concepts that complement each other. One is to work on becoming an addict. The other is to learn to listen to the exercise needs of your own body.

Curious? Stay with me and read on, please.

Ever wonder why it is next to impossible for a person who exercises regularly year in and year out to stop doing it. For me, it will take the loss of a limb or life. But why?

The reason is that exercise causes the release of chemicals called endorphins, which are the body's own naturally occurring opiates or, in other words, our own morphine. These highly addictive endorphins are why we feel good and elated after exercise and sleep better.

If you exercise with some regularity, you give yourself a good chance of getting addicted to these endorphins. Trust me in that this is one healthy addiction you want to get hooked on.

To listen to the exercise needs of your body is not easy and especially at the beginning. You have to be attentive and appreciative of this opiate addiction or the feeling of well-being after exercise. It is then that your body will try talking to you. It will ask you, nudge you and even beg you for more. And you would need to exercise to keep it supplied with endorphins. It will be happy if you comply and not so if you do not.

This silent and subtle conversation with your body is not easy to strike, but once you get it going, the joys are all yours to reap and keep. Over time this keeps getting better with your body telling you how much to exercise, its preferred routines, and when it needs to take a day off.

If you can somehow manage to sneak in and stay in this zone of a perpetual and self-sustaining spiral of regular physical exercise, you shall be living your best life yet, and I guarantee you that.

Good Luck.

BOO

(November 2015, Thanksgiving)

Taking their turn on Halloween, the trick and treating children, those cute little monsters.
And for the rest of the year, creating some real-life freaks, we may have taken upon us.
Here are two very different yet similar scenarios.
One of that angry, disgruntled young man.
Out to settle a score with a gun in hand.
To now becoming routine massacres in schools and places everywhere.
Accepting that in the process, their own death is inevitable.
Often from abused, neglected, and broken homes.
Anything to do with rampant alcohol, loads of infidelity, tons of divorce?
As we shun our responsibilities, could they be paying for our sins?

Or them children of war.
Their cities, their homes, their hopes ripped apart.
Thousands now escaping into the open seas.
Others buying into the extreme ideology to fight back.
Some lured in by the fool's paradise to blow up inside that vest.
State of utter and extreme hopelessness.
Wars begetting wars.
Actioms, reactioms, messsed up, misspellled.
On purpose.
Agreed, this is not the be-all and end-all of the story but aren't many pathologic young minds a result of our adult doings?
And this, my friends, is my point here.
To appreciate and strive for a better world order.
One where we base our actions by their effects on children everywhere.

COMING TOGETHER IS ON YOU, ME, AND EVERYONE

(November 2020,
written as revealed by the woods)

Most human conflicts share in the blame. However, to place all blame on the other side is the fashion, often with no introspection. So, for this political circus and for a change, how about we all accept some blame as in:

Far-left and far-right for stretching the divide. The ones in the middle for conceding such expanse. Mute for staying mute, loud for words without wisdom. The pied-pipers, their nervous followers, their worried enablers, as the next race, for their fate.

We can all accept some failing as in:
The majority because they were a majority, the minority for such an excuse. Weak for staying weak, healthy, not well enough. The heavyweights, Democrats, and Republicans, anything but.

The media for pushing a population into fringes. The educated for not knowing better. The uneducated for not knowing better. Get the drift? For our polarized society, can you and I be any responsible?

Neither angel nor satan, only imperfect, bitter, and human. What would it take to let go of the hate? How about I do it for mine, and you do it for your own sweet sake.

How else can we quit playing God, hand each other a break, another chance, pass around some patience, respect each other's space and presence?

Whereas breaking apart is readily done by a few, coming together is on you, me, and everyone.

The woods are responsible for the content of this message to all people, politicians, FOX, and CNN.

AYLAN

(September 2, 2015, the lifeless body of 3-year-old Syrian boy,
Aylan, washes ashore, trying to escape the war zones
of the Middle East. His picture made global headlines)

Wash away the washed-up Aylan from our conscience
Pretend that it never happened

And somehow undo this stirred up hornet's nest
Anything that helps prevent bursting our bubble

If this is the Arab Spring
It has to get better than this

Or some other galaxy's Armageddon
For ours would need to wait its turn

Dog eat dog
Never on this planet, not on our watch

Shall we gather our pieces and do it better all over again?
For all of them Aylans who are not going to have a picture taken

APPNA PERFECT

(Dec 2017, APPNA is the Association of Physicians
of Pakistani Descent of North America)

It is perfectly all right to

- disregard the smaller alumni and oppositions.
- treat the voter shabby once done running elections.
- vote on regional and alumni lines and not on merit.
- continue to annihilate, belittle, and discourage women leaders on any and all pretext.
- judge this writing not by those participating but by the ones ignoring it.
- try and lead us even if implicated in fraud, convicted, indicted.
- align and divide into man groups and play "who is the bigger king" of all.
- treat the voter rude if they are not supporting y'all.
- assume that all members are idiots and open to abuse.
- quit talking, have yelling matches, bring on lawsuits to settle disputes.
- shine as individuals and underachieve as a group.
- never work across the aisle for the greater good.
- disagree with being disagreeable.
- dream on about our true potential.
- scratch pride, together, greater from our vocabulary.
- continue our ways with apathy, jealousy, animosity.
- against the run of play, keep out qualified women from the BOT,
Wo dahdi bari thee.
Ohdi wari roti ghat gai cee.
- never admit fault, mujhe kyun nikala, never say sorry.
- never join appna, for the glass is half empty.

- ask not what I can do for the organization, ask what the organization can do for me.
- think all Muslim, neglect the minority.
- consider appna as private property.
- think now, my today; forget us, our legacy.
- believe that you own yours truly.

Footnote: In many ways, I find APPNA a microcosm of Pakistan and the larger Muslim world. Good or not so, when I write APPNA, I bare my own self. The object is simple. Encourage, challenge, make better.
This remains a work of satire.

APPNA ELECTIONS 2017

A lone woman is competing this year.
One out of six on the roster.
Trying to break into the upper APPNA echelons.
All lovely people, all friends.
All men Board of Trustees.
All male Executive Committee.
What is the lady thinking?
How dare she!

AMERICAN JOKER

(August 2016)

There's a joker in our midst
Somersaulting, pretending, condescending
Irresponsible, isolating, insulting
Inhumane racist
Dangerously naive and inept
A world-class embarrassment
Arguably the most despised face on the planet
A psychotic volcano staying erupt
Ill-tempered, thin-skinned
There's a joker in our midst

Pass the blame, scare and shame, torch the flame
Declare the endgames open
Championing hate, division, and confusion
Specializing in blunders, one after another
In your face bully, encouraging violence
An egoistic, narcissistic maniac
Disaster in waiting to forever re-happen
Mocking people, calling them names
Utterly, unabashedly, unapologetically, un-American
Here's to a dose of its own medicine
Poor choice of words, such mediocre taste
Passed a mirror and caught a glimpse
There's a joker in our midst

AMERICAN AFGHAN WAR SURGE AND PAKISTAN BASHING

(September 2017, from the
perspective of a Pakistani American)

The Afghan war is going nowhere. Taliban and their support groups, several thousand strong, still run parts of the country and have played the game of patience really well, where the response is measured over decades and centuries, the kind of time NATO and the Americans do not have.

9/11 happened in the year 2001. This is 2017. Look at the map of Afghanistan. Look at the ring of countries surrounding Afghanistan and then the ring surrounding those countries. In Afghanistan today, we, the Americans, are out of time and place and with no endgame in sight. We had it good. We tried to make it better. Now we have neither.

There were lessons from history ignored all along. Lessons from the Vietnam war, the fact that no foreign power has ever ruled over Afghanistan, and the Pashtun mindset. Pashtuns make up the largest portion of the Afghan population, the Taliban, and their allies. My mother was a Pashtun, and I know a thing or two about the culture.

The best analogy of Pashtun psychology though not exactly is the American Rednecks. Conservative, proud of their heritage, seemingly arrogant, heavily armed per capita, warriors, hunters, resilient, stubborn, at times self-destructive with a die-hard and never quit attitude, and I am only scratching the surface. That a four to five figure army of Taliban and the Haqqani network has held off a once six-figure NATO and the American troop presence is what

I am alluding to. That the modern wars run guerilla-style in towns and cities, killing mainly non- participatory populations, are not winnable is what I am talking about.

I would have bought the bashing of Pakistan if it was on a joyride in the last decade all the time while America was grinding its teeth. The reality is anything but. There was a time a few years back when Lahore, the city I grew up in, a bustling metropolis of over 11 million, where a lot of my family still lives, was getting sabotaged by regular terror attacks and bombings. I can never forget when one of my relatives told me that when they leave home in the morning, they are not sure how many would be back that evening. What we as Americans need to understand is the direct and indirect devastation our actions and these wars have brought upon a lot of this World's population who had absolutely nothing to do with the falling of those towers on that ill-fated day in September.

To blame Pakistan for the Afghan conundrum is like blaming the cornerman for the result of a boxing match, a cornerman who has himself received a lot of blows during. Pakistan has had its own love-hate relationship with these groups, has been ravaged by terrorism from these groups, and, of course and rightly so, is going to watch its own interest first and find its own mechanism for dealing with these groups. It has had some success lately, as evidenced by a significant decrease in the number of terror attacks there.

Please understand that in the modern world of easy access and news sharing, one person's terrorist may be another's Robin Hood. Even our adversaries and terrorists of today were our comrades and allies in the war against the Soviet Union, a war where Pakistan helped America across the finish line. While we in America call out others for terrorism, there are those who consider us the same. Gone are the days of American moral superiority. These long, drawn-out wars and especially the Iraq war with its massive casualties and all that for what again, have ripped the topsoil off the American moral high ground.

And then there is the philosophy of war. In a heavyweight vs. lightweight contest, there is only so much sympathy, and for so long, the heavyweight is going to get even if the original reasoning for the conflict was correct. The heavyweight is more powerful, has more options and thus more responsibility and thus more blame to share and especially when the conflict keeps going on and on and on. Remember, human instinct usually favors the underdog in a contest. No wonder today America is left holding the hot potato with its associated cost and consequences almost all by itself, and I can see where President Trump is coming from in calling out NATO and the UN on this.

Let the local dynamics play and sort it out as painful as it may be in the short term. The long-term, tenable solutions have to come from within, and the best American influence is not by force but by example.

Open them schools in Afghanistan and then some more. Persistently and passionately educate the children of our enemies and then some more. Leave behind loads and loads of books and pencils, blackboard and chalk. How hard can this be? Is it more expensive than 17 years of war?

While we are at it, please fix the year-round potholes on my way to work in Wisconsin and give us all Americans better health care. Yes, we do need money here at home. Please.

As a physician, I live by, "First do no harm" dogma every single day. I came to America not because it had the strongest army but because it was the most caring, generous, and advanced society on this planet. Fight these wars with better ideas, better alternatives, better opportunities, better modernity, better sharing, better living, and better of all and everything good there is. This is the America I know and live in, and this is when the city on the hill shines its best.

AMERICA'S GUN VIOLENCE, A CURSE, OR GOD'S RETRIBUTION?

(February 2018)

On Thursday the 24th of September 2015, Pope Francis addressed the Joint Session of the United States Congress and said this,

"Being at the service of dialogue and peace also means being truly determined to minimize and, in the long term, to end the many armed conflicts throughout our world. Here we have to ask ourselves: Why are deadly weapons being sold to those who plan to inflict untold suffering on individuals and society? Sadly, the answer, as we all know, is simply for money: money that is drenched in blood, often innocent blood. In the face of this shameful and culpable silence, it is our duty to confront the problem and to stop the arms trade."

I have read these lines over and over, thinking that today in America, we are all but helpless to stop the killing of our own on our turf.
Is this a curse coming home to roost?
Is this God's retribution upon us?
Listen to the Holy man, and you decide for yourself.

AMERICA YOU BEAUTY

(April 2018)

Father was in his eighties and more recently looking his age, and something else was not right. He was more short of breath, his ankles were getting swollen, and he was anemic. Being his only son and an ocean and a continent away, this was a nightmare in the works. What if something happens to him while he was away, how would he manage, what would I do, were the ever lingering fears.

Father would typically spend the summer months with us here in the USA on his visitor visa and go back to Lahore, Pakistan, for the winters to live by himself. With my mother and brother already past this world, no immediate family was living with him.

Father was visiting with us here in the USA, and the credit for making the call goes to Farah, my wife. He cannot live by himself; we cannot let him go back, he should stay with us, she said. We talked to him, and he agreed. There were unanswered questions; we were in uncharted territory.

Further testing confirmed heart failure, colon cancer, weak kidneys, and transfusion-dependent anemia. To the US immigration, I would forward these reports and mention that his conditions are terminal, I am his physician and only son and would request that father be allowed to stay under my care here in the US.

Each time he would get a six-month extension of his visitor visa status. The University hospital in town provided compassionate care. Dear friends, family, neighbors, and all pitched in and helped. He genuinely loved them, and they loved him back. Father knew what was coming, was very comfortable with it, and would spend most of his time praying, a content old man getting ready for his end and the hereafter.

Father passed away in November of 2009, his last few weeks in hospice care were a miracle. He stayed with us for his last years of life and is buried not far from where we live.

A few weeks later, we received a further six-month extension of his stay from the Immigration services. I wrote them back, updating them about his demise and thanking them profusely.

Fast forward to 2018, where in the middle of the American debate on gun violence, mass shootings, and mental health, I wrote "My brother" and posted it on "The Moderate Voice," a broad-based Internet news outlet.

Soon afterward, I received an email from Joe Gandelman, the Editor-In-Chief of the site, asking, "If you have a photo of your brother, send it to me, and I can put it on the post." I found this photo with my mother, father, and brother and sent it to Joe, who then posted the picture with the article and featured it at the top of the site and here is the link, http://themoderatevoice.com/my-brother/

I have never met or spoken to Joe, our introduction and interactions have only been through our writings and emails.

Now America picks up a lot of flak for its shortcomings, but someone has to give it credit for its soul and the good it brings to the table.

With a written word, a picture, a gravesite, and many considerate people, my family above, is now and forever, right here with me and a part of the American story.

I get to see a lot of this side of America, perhaps because I live among everyday Americans, for this is the better American essence, and this is what America does best.

AMERICA IS ITS PEOPLE

(September 2016)

We smile at each other for no apparent reason.
We hold doors open without knowing the other person.
We cherish our way of life, our freedoms.
A nation of immigrants, we are The Americans.
We debate passionately, we disagree.
We teach our young decency.
We attract the best from all over the planet.
To an equal for all society.
The world's largest economy.
Where anything is possible.
Here skies don't limit us.
We sit atop the World Giving Index.
And the Research and Development spending list.
The biggest contributor to the United Nations.
The most decorated nation in the Olympics.
By Holly, we create magic on the screen.
Microsoft, Boeing, IBM, Google.
Facebook, Twitter, Amazon, Apple.
Tracks on Mars, footprints on the moon.
Never by chance, not a coincidence.
Our substance, this eminence, is for a reason.
All for that brilliantly written word.
We the People.
For our Constitution.

A VERY AMERICAN THING

(January 2017)

A declared war on our minds and bodies
A society struggling to come to grips with
In our face, eyes shut, we can own this
Morbid Obesity is a very American thing
The rest of the World just ain't this big

A GIFT, EARLY IN THE PANDEMIC

(April 2020)

A world in lockdown, I step out every day to fight an enemy I cannot see. I arm myself by giving to those worse hit than me.
I wear my destiny and well wishes and acts of kindness such as these.
A gift of hand-sewn caps and masks from my neighbor, thank you Boni Kuenzi.

38-YEAR-OLD JACINDA ARDERN, A MESSIAH AND A WOMAN

(March 2019)

Even before the Christchurch, New Zealand Mosque massacre
The thought had crossed my mind more than once
Prostrate in Friday congregation in any US mosque,
we are all praying ducks
I have seen the New Zealand massacre video
Seen the worshippers take bullets, coil away, and die without resistance
No different perhaps from any other Man eat Mankind
except this one was broadcast live
For a few days in solemn,
the entire world came together as one
Overwhelming grace and kindness, though,
won the moment
A country called New Zealand, a Messiah by the name of Jacinda Ardern
They all pitched in big at the love end

32 EXPATRIATES, PAKISTANIS, AND INDIANS AGAINST A NUCLEAR STANDOFF

(March 2019)

For Pakistanis and Indians everywhere and in the US, in a week of seesaw diplomacy and unsettling war games.

I am nervous.

An ongoing cricket tournament in Madison, Wisconsin, USA, where Indians and Pakistanis mix up and play.

Though I was nervous with more questions than answers, more doubts than convictions.

Not for the game but for the gamesmanship.

Would we still come together to play, or cancel and stay, in our respective bubbles?

And just like that, the night came and passed, we did gather and play, all trying and going out of their way, to be more gracious, more generous.

Acutely aware of our global citizenship, this one big mother village, our interdependence.

32 expatriates, Pakistanis, and Indians, against the odds, playing cricket over war, choosing team play, and maintaining discourse.

Talking with a bat and a ball, we played for peace, yes peace for all.

1.8 BILLION VILLAINS

(November 2017, President Trump
tweets anti-Muslim videos)

Oops, we got busted again, I hate to admit it.
By who else than our very own President.
As he retweets the far-right anti-Muslim videos.
So under no duress, I am going to confess.
As I am running out of ways to react.
I mean all us Muslims, all 1.8 billion.
We had conspired with Kim Jong-un.
Who agreed to provide cover with his rocket launches.
While we would continue with our evil ways.
1.8 billion had agreed upon and signed off on those incidents which Trump mentions.
Yes, I remember Mr. Islam in attendance.
All 1.8 billion involved in some form of terrorism.
Just as all white folks are guilty of Donald J Trump.
And all brown people for having the brown skin pigment.
Just can't keep getting caught like this.
We are 1.8 billion villains.
Pretty soon, no one would want to live with us.
Goddamn it.
Imagine 1.8 billion shopping for a new planet.

Footnote: This is a work of satire.

www.ingramcontent.com/pod-product-compliance
Lightning Source LLC
Chambersburg PA
CBHW030907080526
44589CB00010B/181